Gro Elisabeth Walle is a Norwegian author, artist, dreamworker and healer. Gro was born in Cameroon, Africa in 1951, where her parents were missionaries. When she was 15, the family moved to Norway. Gro became the mother of three children. With a higher education in fine art and teaching she taught and promoted her art successfully. Her life went down a new path when she was divorced. Sick and depressed, she was led to the teaching of healing and self-development. Her passion for dreams, signs and symbols became her new focus of studies as she developed a special skill in connecting intuitive art – and dreamwork. She gave speeches, workshops and wrote articles in renowned magazines, appearing on national TV.

At the age of 58, she left Norway and travelled to the USA and Mexico and eventually wrote *I Dreamt I Was Flying*, which is a testimony of how following dreams and signs can bring you home to your true self.

I dedicate my book to my children, Mikal, Jan Mathias and June,
my light and joy.

Gro Elisabeth Walle

I Dreamt I Was Flying

A True Story About a Magical Journey
of Healing, Where Dreams and
Signs Gave Direction

AUSTIN MACAULEY PUBLISHERS™

LONDON * CAMBRIDGE * NEW YORK * SHARJAH

A CIP catalogue record for this title is available from the British Library.

ISBN 9781398430938 (Paperback)
ISBN 9781398430945 (ePub e-book)

www.austinmacauley.com

First Published 2022
Austin Macauley Publishers Ltd®
1 Canada Square
Canary Wharf
London
E14 5AA

20230927

Besides friends and family who encouraged me along the way, my Norwegian publisher Ingebjørg Nesheim was a patient and invaluable midwife. My mother Lilly Walle contributed in an important way also. A childhood friend amazingly appeared on the scene when I needed help with the translation into English. Samara, a beautiful daughter of a dear friend of mine, came to my rescue when I needed it the most. Then my dear friend, PJ Mann, helped me with corrections in the final stage of the editing of my English writing. That turned out to be a big and important task! Thank you from the bottom of my heart to you all!

I am also deeply grateful to Austin Macauley Publishers for bringing this book out to the world. Healers, authors, and guides from all around the world helped me find illustrations and words to knowledge that I had forgotten, although deep inside had known all along.

Table of Contents

I stopped trying to fashion a life with just the right job, personal relationships, and projects, as if there were a simple mathematical equation for happiness. Instead, I learned to operate from a higher perspective and open up to wider definitions of joy and success. Then I discovered the power to create a different story for the world and myself. Only then could I let go of the stories I kept telling myself...which were trapping me in a limited existence.

– Alberto Villoldo,
The Four Insights

Introduction

The future belongs to those who believe in the beauty of dreams.

– Eleanor Roosevelt

I was eight years old. It was Saturday afternoon and the air was heavy with rain. I was standing in the courtyard outside the boarding school, where my siblings and I lived. We were in a town called Ngaoundéré, in northern Cameroon, about a day's travel from home, through the warm African savanna.

It was months since we had last seen our parents. The longing for them had shifted to a quiet, sad acceptance. I stood there, smelling the air like an animal. Something was different this Saturday. I had this strange feeling my dad was somewhere close. It was rainy season and the roads could be hazardous. They were often washed away by the rain or the car could get stuck in deep mud holes, so we did not expect our parents to visit at this time of the year. If my Dad were to suddenly show up now, it would have been very unusual. I stood quietly and listened intently. Something out there was drawing my attention so strongly that I blocked everything else out. All my senses were wide open and receptive. Some time passed and suddenly I heard our car and excitedly shouted to my siblings, "Dad is coming! Dad is coming!" Time passed, and nothing happened. There was no indication of any car, but *I knew it was out there somewhere* – not far away. I was convinced I could both hear and 'smell' it! Finally, we could all hear it and were ecstatically happy! Thinking back now, it was the most intense joy I can remember experiencing as a child. I didn't think any more about this strange experience where I seemed to know what was to happen before it did. It seemed so natural to me.

Experiencing my intuition at work was not something weird here. Africa supported and nourished all such gifts and I experienced premonitions a few more times during my stay at the boarding school. But then, my imagination created what I wished for. I heard the car without anything happening. The disappointment hurt and I began to doubt this quiet little voice. Then it weakened even more as we moved from intuitive Africa to frigid Norway, a country ruled by the mental, rational and safe. My confidence in this small quiet inner voice was tucked away, together with my power and radiance. Like the bright African sun I left behind, these aspects of me seemed unwelcome in the cold, dark North.

Many years later, I had a dream where I was almost forced, by two of my deceased ancestors, to write this book and share my miraculous experiences and journey through life. I understood I could not refuse. *I Dreamt I was Flying* is a testimony to how we all can dream our life into a new reality. We are much greater than our sensible and fearful minds dare to dream.

After many years of working as an artist, teacher, art therapist and spiritual counsellor, I will not refer to any of my clients in this book; instead, I have chosen to use my own life as the backdrop to all the dreams and miraculous encounters. All the signs and symbols I was given, were road-signs for me to follow. To be able to interpret dreams, signs and synchronicities, one needs to see them in the context of one's current situations. Therefore, I am sharing the story of my journey. It is a *gift* I am supposed to bring forward.

Our dreams are doorways to our higher self and the higher realms where our guides and helpers of the *light* can connect with us. I discovered the Universe was just waiting to help me when my life forced me 'to let go and let God'. I was guided every step by signs, dreams and synchronicities. I just had to allow myself to see them and open my heart to my inner voice again that had been buried deep within me. I started to listen to the voice of nature again. It's speaking to us all the time, always telling us to say 'Yes' to our heart, our inner light. Nature never says no. It just turns toward what it wants. It always says *Yes* to the sun.

Like a *Caterpillar*, we are coming into this reality to explore life on the material level, struggling through highs and lows, experiences and choices. Then comes the time to process all experiences in stillness at the deepest levels of our being. In a *Cocoon,* we go through the process of releasing, transforming and redefining who we are. At last, we are ready to let go of our pain story and experience who we really are, and the beauty that lies within.

As a *Butterfly* we are free to fly and serve the world with our beauty, gifted by *Spirit*, as the *Sun* shines through our wings. As most of us do, I had forgotten my power and hidden the true joy deep inside because I was afraid of its immense beauty and strength.

I have had a different childhood than most Norwegian children, being born and raised in Africa, but my adult life in Norway seemed normal, although challenging. Later, I went to the US to experience how to dream big and believe I deserve the gifts of life. The great contrast between these continents was often difficult to handle given my sensitivity. Still, I believe many will resonate with the many ups and downs, and the chaotic dance of victories, defeats and losses I am about to describe. I stumbled, got back on my feet and stumbled again until one day I remained down, unable to get back up again. The crisis hit me hard and pushed me outside of my comfort zone. It woke me up. Everything I encountered, confirmed I am not alone on this earthly journey. Life is safer, larger, more magical and way more beautiful than I could imagine.

I discovered I was part of a much larger and beautiful world-loom: *Africa gave me the gifts of intuition and creativity, the countries of the North gave me the gifts of analytical thinking and willpower, and the States gave me support and faith that my dreams could be manifested.* We all are connected to everything around us – mirroring each other all the time. We are supposed to fulfil each other by being the best that we can be, because we are *One Body*. This book is no academic documentation of dreams, nor is it an attempt to explain the reasons why we dream. It's not a manual to explain dream work or the interpretation of symbols. We all can develop our individual emotional association to pictures and symbols. But while I tell my story, I refer to respected sources and the collective ancient knowledge that has inspired me. And although the dreams shared are personal, I leave myself open to the fact that many of them might reflect something beyond the very personal some truths that are happening on a shared universal level. I believe we share this collective consciousness more than we realise, so I trust many will recognise themselves in much of what I experienced.

Hopefully, this book, as a sharing of my own magical journey, will inspire others to seek and find understanding and help in their own dreams and daily small and big events. I also hope this book will be an inspiration to you who might feel you are trapped in your personal circumstances, as I thought I was. It is all about changing our perceptions.

Chapter 1
Bandon

The divine purpose of your life is often experienced in your consciousness as a glimpse of something that is too good to be true.

– Florence S. Shinn

"I did it! Can you believe that I actually made it?" I was ecstatic as I walked towards the airplane. Fifty-eight years old and free to travel. I was ready for an extended stay in the United States. Half a year earlier, I had been on a shorter exploratory trip to the West Coast. That is when I discovered Bandon in Oregon and this is where I was now headed.

In Norway, I had everything I needed, except good health and joy. I had to escape this sober, respectable and controlled atmosphere for a while. Life in Norway had made me sick. I needed to breathe new air and so I sold my flat, gave away everything I owned and left! With two suitcases and some loose idea of what I wanted to do, I boarded the plane, ready to build a new life with fresh, happy memories. I was convinced the Universe was supporting and guiding me. A small voice inside was starting to cheer cautiously.

My children were now grown and settled, and they had given me their blessing for this adventure. I chose to trust that what was best for me was also best for my children, and for my old mother who was left behind.

Six months earlier, I had travelled by train across the continent to Portland, Oregon. One day, while visiting a small shop I had the impulse to ask the young couple working there if they knew of a nice place for me to stay for my next extended trip the US. My preference was to go a little further south on the West Coast of Oregon. The young couple told me they had heard of a place called Bandon. They had never been there themselves, but they heard it was a beautiful and quiet place. Somehow the name resonated with me, but I couldn't find it on the map. Still I stopped looking for other options. I felt at peace and enjoyed the rest of the train ride down the West Coast without giving it further thought, realising I still had to return to Norway to sell the flat before I could afford to plan for that longer stay.

After three months of travels during this first visit and experiencing this amazing country, the time had come to return to Norway. I took a quick detour to New Jersey on the east coast to visit my friends Mona and David. David pulled out a map which he thought would be big and detailed enough to include Bandon. The map was in front of me on the table, but the writing was so small that I needed glasses to see. I was so impatient that I let my finger glide over the map to 'try to find it' when my finger stopped at a spot jutting out from the coast south in Oregon. *Maybe it's there*! I thought and ran to fetch my glasses. I was very curious to see where my finger had stopped. And there it was – Bandon, clear as day! Well, that settled it, I had found my place, no doubt! We carefully explored all the information we could find about Bandon. The coat of arms was a lighthouse! We also read that you can see the whales from shore when they migrate during spring and fall. I had a strange sensation when I read this. Earlier, I had a dream about a beautiful place on the West Coast, where I supposedly was living and where whales were passing by. I really hadn't thought so much about this dream until now. I returned to Norway and sold my home. Suddenly, it wasn't a difficult decision to make. But to sell the apartment at that time in May 2008 was risky. Very few were buying. Still, I contacted my real-estate agent, a young Muslim lady and hoped for the best. Somehow, I had peace that all would work out just fine. I got along very well with the real-estate agent and when I told her that I often meditate, she wanted to learn too, and I was happy to help her. I guided her into the quiet, holy place we all have inside whether we are Muslims, Christians or non-religious. She was astonished to discover the profound effect meditation had and asked me to please help her sister and mother who suffered from severe anxiety. I was happy to help. Two weeks later, my agent had sold my flat above the expected rate.

One of the last days before departure, I went to visit one of my brothers, only a ten-minute train ride away. While sitting on the train, I suddenly felt uneasy and closed my eyes, breathing deeply. "Please give me a last confirmation that I have chosen the right place to go." I sighed. Then I let go of the concern, feeling sure that the answer would come when the time was right. I sat next to a lady engrossed in her reading. I usually never peek over peoples' shoulders to check what they are reading when I travel, but this time I did. 'Bandon was magical,' I read – the sentence seemingly popping out from the middle of the page! I heaved a sigh of relief and the sensation of deep gratitude spread throughout my body. I was very impressed and had to smile thinking of the quick and creative answer I had received. Bandon is a very small place that few people know about, even in Oregon, and there I was in Norway on the opposite side of the world reading about it. And then, six months later, I was boarding the plane, finally on my way to this strange small place on the coast of Oregon. This was the start of a beautiful adventure I never would have expected.

After 12 hours on the plane, we landed in San Francisco. I wanted to stay here a couple of days and get adjusted before moving on and taking the bus up north to Bandon. I whispered a silent prayer that I would feel welcome when I stepped out of the plane. I had never been here before and did not know anyone. I picked up my luggage and started walking towards the entrance when a nicely dressed man walked up to me. He asked if I was going to the centre of town and if I was interested in sharing a car, half price? I politely declined remembering some unpleasant experiences with pirate taxis in Paris. But when he explained another couple was also traveling in the same car, I agreed to go with them. Outside a long black and shiny limousine was waiting. We met up with the couple, greeted each other cheerfully and boarded. Beautifully polished wine glasses were lined up on the shelf above us and there were lots of twinkling lights in the window. It seemed the Christmas decorations were still out, even though it was now April! *We might as well enjoy the ride,* I thought, as we laughed and giggled with childlike delight enjoying the extravagance of our surroundings. We did feel special. Through the open skylight the stars were twinkling from a dark, clear sky. *That is promising!* I thought, thanking the angels or whoever orchestrated such a wonderful welcome. Something or someone was looking after me.

San Francisco filled me with warmth, colours and inspiring artistic experiences. After a couple of days enjoying this energising atmosphere—food for the soul—I headed north to Oregon. I thought the trip would take about nine hours, but I must have still suffered from jet lag as I realised I had misread the ticket and the bus ride took nineteen hours! Still it all went smoothly. I took in all the impressions from this new and multifaceted country. Norwegians use public transport a lot, but here a white elderly lady with a backpack traveling alone by train and bus was out of the ordinary. I was met with interest and respect and often ended up in interesting conversations, especially with young people. They listened to thoughts and experiences I shared while I received good advice and information about the places I was going to visit. Every encounter seemed important and the Universe was lovingly guiding and watching over me.

When I finally arrived in Bandon, I knew I was in the right place. This is where I was going to stay over the next six months. "How come you ended up in Bandon?" asked a shop owner I struck up a conversation with.

"It's a miracle!" was all I could answer.

"Yes that is often how people find us. This is a magical place!" he answered with a smile.

One night, not long after I had settled in a big and wonderful house in Bandon, I had an upsetting dream (Chapter 1: Dream nr 1; Rescue my baby). I dreamt I had let the man I had been married to, take care of my baby. He had wrapped it in so many blankets that the baby could not breathe, and he put it in a drawer. I desperately picked up the baby from the drawer and unwrapped it. I was so ashamed that I had let this man take care of the baby.

Waking up, I felt very unsettled. Something needed saving, but what? I took time to sense the feelings I had during the dream. I could not let myself get scared by this feeling. Fear is rooted in ego; it fights changes. I had to find peace to be able to interpret this dream. Closing my eyes and breathing deeply, I let myself slowly be led into a quiet space. I focused fully on my breathing as it led me past the fear and into the silence. Here I could face the dream again. I examined each facet of the dream and noted what it wanted to tell me: air is essential. Symbolically air represents thought, communication and life-force. I had wrapped up and put away my dream and tucked it away in a drawer. Now, I knew it was time to pull it out, take off the layers of protections, and confront everything that had prevented me from being happy.

The man in the dream represented the active and mental part of me. My ex-husband was born in the astrological sign of Libra which represents the Air element and symbolises mental energy. Creativity, beauty and harmony are potential gifts of the sign of Libra. Libra is also associated with media and are therefore represents the communicator and mediator. All gifts to be developed. But Libra's shadow side tends to sweep things under the carpet, or "put things away in a drawer" rather than having a confrontation.

Libra's shadow side is that it tends to 'sweep things under the carpet,' or 'put things away in a drawer', rather than having a confrontation. Fear of confrontation is the weak aspect of Libra and therefore often delays important and difficult choices and decisions.

I had wrapped up the process and delayed the work on the book I knew I was supposed to write. The baby symbolised the project. Now was the time to unwrap it and give it life. I was thankful for the reminder. It became clear that I was not only here on vacation.

I pulled out all those journals I had brought along. Here I had jotted down dreams, thoughts and experiences collected through many years. I was ready to put into words all that had manifested as physical symptoms and unconscious problems. I wanted to see and understand the greater context of my life and find my way out of the pain story into my life purpose and greatest potential. I wanted to reveal the gift of it all, and I was ready to write it in a book. I now understood I would be guided and supported in this process.

The house I was offered in Bandon was big, beautiful and unbelievably cheap. Here I could safely work in peace. Everything was facilitated just perfectly. The address was 630 June Ave. My daughter is named June and my life number is nine, the root-sum of 630. A perfect synchronicity!

Larva:

In this life, my journey begins as a caterpillar struggling through the first level of life, on the 'Red Road of the Rainbow-bridge'. In this level, I learn to understand the physical world. I become strengthened by all the challenges and obstacles I find in myself and around me.

The experiences have been absorbed; the learning harvested. I am ready for the next level, all in line with my Divine Life-plan.

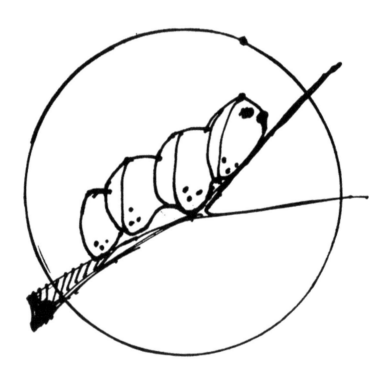

Chapter 2
Life's Contrasts

I am a citizen of the world and my nationality is Goodwill.

– Socrates

Looking back at the bigger picture of my past, I see everything is meant for growth. The obstacles are just contrasting experiences to wake us up. We are just collecting knowledge and everything has a purpose, even the pain. When I was willing to see and listen, I was given signs and dreams for support and guidance. I was shown the shadow is as important as the light.

Here I was in Bandon, free from any expectations and old bonds. I could give myself my own undivided focus. As I am easily distracted, this place and time was perfect for my inner journey. One of my first nights in Bandon, I had a strange dream (Chapter 2: Dream nr 2: Meeting with elephants). I dreamt I was going into a big forest with beautiful, tall trees. Suddenly, a huge elephant came charging. I was so scared that I ran onto a path that appeared to the left and suddenly I stood at a clearing where there were several elephants standing in a row. They were not as big and frightening as the first one, but I was still scared as there were many of them. The elephants all stood on their hind legs, trunks extended and saluting me with impressive, loud trumpet-like sounds. I stood there, surprised and respectfully watching the show. Then I was led further down the path to the left and came to a large and beautiful hall with a fantastic display of food. I could help myself with whatever I wanted from a table with wonderfully delightful desserts. I discovered I was wearing a gorgeous long, blue gown.

The elephant symbolises the grounding of spirit and represents a wise, safe force. Happiness often accompanies the elephant, they say. The elephant is also known to have an impressively good memory and carry memories throughout their lifetime. The forest symbolises my subconscious. I understood that I must make the inward journey and dare to face every 'memory' that appears on my path.

The desserts represent something that will come to me later…as a reward if I dared to make this journey, I thought. I would also have to grow into this queenly energy: the blue colour of the gown was a symbol of strength and wisdom.

Close to the house where I lived there was a row of huge old trees. Their trunks were smooth and grey and could resemble the legs of an elephant. The trees were planted a long time ago to protect the inhabitants in Bandon from the unceasing winds blowing through this small coastal town. I was comforted and encouraged by this dream to trust I would be helped, protected, and rewarded throughout the process of my inner work and on my journey.

I opened my journals and started to pull on the threads of my stories. It was easier to look back into these memories from a distance. The bigger picture was becoming clearer. I could now see I had been pushed, supported, and guided by 'It All' along my whole life. When an artist is building a picture, she must always use contrasting colors to bring the picture to life. Otherwise, it easily becomes a flat and lifeless picture. The frictions make us react and grow.

In one of my journals, I found this dream (Chapter 2: Dream nr 3: The path of contrasts) about the contrasts of life. At the time I had this dream, I was living in Norway and was newly divorced. What I was experiencing at this time made me quite sick. Both my mind and body were feeling the pain. In the dream, I was walking on a path through a forest. This path was covered with dark green and crimson crystals. They were sharp and it hurt to step on them, but I thought they were so beautiful and picked up a few to put in a kerchief I had brought along. There was a big flat stone at the side of the path, and it was covered with the same crystals. They were arranged as a round ornament with strange symbols. I brought the big stone along although it was very heavy. I had a feeling this was important. But I was honestly despairing that I had to walk this painful although beautiful path. Next, I woke up.

Crystals signify old and pure knowledge. Red and green are contrasting colours and represent polarities in the heart. It is painful to walk on the path of contrasts. Still as humans in this third dimension, we seem unable to learn except through pain! In our search for balance and harmony, we unconsciously explore the polarities. To create harmony in my life, I needed to learn how to unite and balance the extremes and contrasts in myself. I had to seek to find the balance between thought and feeling to create harmony in my life. Everything had to be integrated through my heart. This was to become the most difficult but also most important lesson. A couple of years later, I learned the round symbol on the stone slab was the shamanic wheel of life, representing the four directions and elements in our universe. It shows the road to harmony from the contrast we experience and teaches us how everything is linked together. Everything must balance through the centre of the wheel of life which represents our hearts, and the entrance of cosmos. I knew nothing about this wheel of life when I had the dream in Norway.

I am continually surprised by the fact that my dreams often show me things of which I have no prior knowledge. The knowledge is in us all, but it must be awakened and made conscious. In this dream, I received a hint of where my path would lead, long before I was ready to walk it.

In the peace of Bandon, I dived safely into my memories and my thoughts. I am a citizen of the world exploring the mysteries of existence. Some called me a Christian mystic. That was okay. At the age of 45, when everything around me had collapsed, I had asked Kaja Finne, my Norwegian therapist, "Why was I born in Africa and had to move to Norway?" I was standing at a crossroad, bewildered as to which way to choose.

"You were supposed to experience the contrasts," she answered. "And to bring the African sunshine to Norway," she added with a friendly smile. There it was again – the African Sun within me. I had tucked it away for so long. Kaja then asked me the fundamental question: "Do you know who you are, Gro?" That released a surprisingly strong reaction and it was painful to recognise that I did not know. I realised, as tears were running down my cheeks, one of my deepest longings was to understand who I am. I later thought maybe she saw 'who I am' and decided to push a button to awaken a sleeping awareness in me. At this point, I started a long and demanding study of self-realisation. I am happy that I did not know how painful, long, and costly this journey would be. I had to climb the heights to see things in perspective and go down into the dark to explore the hidden. I had to be an outsider to receive insight and dare to be alone to make friends with myself. I also had to go behind the curtain to realise all the different roles I was playing, often without even knowing I was doing so. I wanted to unveil what had created the person I thought I was – but who I discovered was not the real me.

Solitude is used to teach us how to live with other people. Rage is used to show us the infinite value of peace. Boredom is used to underline the importance of adventure and spontaneity. Silence is used to teach us to use words responsibly. Tiredness is used so that we can understand the value of waking up. Illness is used to underline the blessing of good health. Fire is used to teach us about water. Earth is used so that we can understand the value of air. Death is used to show us the importance of life.

– Paulo Coelho

In hindsight, I could see how I was led to cultures and environments where I gained experiences of contrast that stimulated growth and greater insight. The world proved to be infinitely larger, more diverse, and immensely more beautiful than I had imagined.

I discovered the same on my inward journey. I learned the universe was filled with expansive creative power and we all are a part of this. This is the force that inspires us to continue to grow our awareness. I have learned the spirit that is in everything 'speaks' and shows us what we need to know and understand. I just had to learn to listen, see and recognise it. Through generations of scepticism towards the metaphysical, extrasensory, and the teachings about our inner universe, many of us have lost this valuable knowledge. We, therefore, live in a divided world. The split between mind and spirit has started a war within us. To regain peace, these two worlds will have to unite. Opposites want to unite and find their way home, and everything must unite through the heart. The whole world and all its conflicts and dividedness are mirrored within me.

In my quest for answers and understanding the bigger picture, I had to go further back in time to find the origin of my pain-story. The path of contrasts I had chosen to walk, made me want to understand the reasons, because I knew my past had affected my choices for the future. I had to embrace and reveal the dark to be able to understand and embrace the light within me. The picture I wanted to paint would need to contain every colour and all the shades of dark and light to be a unified and true picture. My childhood in Africa was filled with colourful contrasts of dark and light, and joy and pain. It was an important backdrop to my journey into the future. Our body and mind carry the remembrance of all our experiences and that affects our beliefs about who we think we are.

Chapter 3
Africa and the Intuitive Child

There are only two ways to live life. One is as though nothing is a miracle. The other is as though everything is a miracle. I believe in the latter.

– Albert Einstein

I remember as a child, living far from home and feeling alone, my dream was to create a paradise on Earth where we all could live safe and peaceful together. I would have visions of this in dreams and sometimes they would appear in the quiet when I was out in nature. Many would call me a dreamer, but they said it made sense since I was to become an artist because I was good at drawing. It was accepted and understood. But the reality was I didn't know what an artist was supposed to be like and therefore had no aspirations of becoming one. I just liked to draw. Our small, isolated community out in the bush in Africa gave no indication of the diversity of choices so far in the future on a different continent.

I was just seven years old and dreaming of preaching for people, not like a priest in church, but for people at large, anywhere they could be found. I wanted to communicate about how we, as humans, should treat each other and how together we could create a paradise. Already at seven, this was my secret dream. But I could not find the words to express it, so it remained a silent dream.

Africa is under the astrological sign of Pisces that is a playful, emotional, intuitive, and creative energy. It is 'the feet of Mother Earth'. People are sensitive and emotional and close to their ancestral predisposition. Here, I learned everything in nature is alive and has a voice. I learned to 'read the signs.'

I was the oldest of seven children. My sister was six and I was seven years old when we were sent to a boarding school about a day's journey from our home. My other siblings also joined us when they came of age. We returned home to our family only twice a year due to a lack of adequate infrastructure and bad roads. This deeply affected us, of course. Many years later, the hurts came to the surface and could no longer be suppressed or denied. They erupted in both physical and psychological symptoms. Strange how much a child can endure. But the body never forgets.

They call Africa the cradle of the world. It is situated on the southern hemisphere and represents the intuitive and creative child. The gifts of this continent were big and strong. The sun was warm and bright, but the night was dark and cold. The summer was hot and dry, and the winter was wet and fertile. It is a continent of contrasts really. Everything has two sides and one can find a gift in every situation. For us children, our circumstances made us independent and strong. We also found a certain freedom in this lifestyle, as we had more space to express ourselves than if we had lived under our parents' protective and watchful eyes. But care, validation and love were in short supply throughout our childhood. We internalised this lack and thought it was the norm.

We felt like Africans deep down and we loved Africa. Cameroon is situated right beneath the equator, and at midday the sun is in zenith. We only experienced two seasons, the rainy and dry season, and the rainy season often surprised us when dark clouds suddenly rolled in over the savanna followed by strong pouring rain. After a cloudburst, the sun would reappear and give life to everything. The dry savanna that seemed dead for several months miraculously came back to life. The contrasts were magic.

Cameroon is half the size of Norway and at the time we lived there had about the same number of inhabitants. Still 150 different tribal languages were spoken in this relatively small country. We learned a tribe-language called *Mbum* and spoke it long before we learned to speak Norwegian. As we started school, we invented new words to replace Norwegian words that seemed foreign to us. Our Norwegian teachers were understanding and obliging, but I became vulnerable when returning to Norway and it was obvious that my Norwegian was inadequate.

The boarding school was in a town called Ngaoundere. It was in the north, surrounded by savanna and a mountain rage. We simply called it "the mountains". Its landforms concealed many secrets that only we the children knew. There were rock formations creating secret passageways, and caves and tunnels to explore. One time, I remember finding a leopard's tail deep inside a cave. It was both scary and exciting to think that maybe some big animals had been fighting right there one dark night. I picked up the tail and quickly crawled out. You never knew what could be hiding back there in the darkness. I looked at these huge rocks and boulders on top of each other. Some were perfectly square and so large they could not have been placed there by humans, I thought. It was very mysterious to us.

There was a small river flowing along the mission compound. There was lots of activity along these banks during the rainy season. Otters played on certain stretches of the river and I stayed away from them. I had learned from the Africans that otters were scary, magical creatures and not to be trusted. I believed them. We found secret places in the tall grass where we also sometimes could find big beautiful lilies. The adults had to ask us if they wanted some for a party, as we were very secretive about these spots.

There were times when our lives were brimming with excitement and fun, but there were also contrasting painful emotions at the boarding school. We learned to use humour to vent out frustration and sadness. Africans are good at this, laughing in the face of sorrow! We made our own stage and acted out our vulnerability. We put together skits where we caricatured the adults and made fun of all our sad experiences. We laughed through afternoons and evenings when we found ourselves alone at the boarding school when the other families went on family outings and picnics. My siblings and I were now too many to be included, and our parents were too far away to be able to keep up with what was happening in our lives. We laughed and made fun of the fact no one understood, but at night the tears could not be held back any longer. The night concealed our tears and our pillows softened our cries.

We developed our empathic side through our experiences. We learned to share. I remember one time, when Dad came on a surprise visit and brought two large green apples for us to share. Most likely they were terribly expensive, bought in one of the few shops in town. These were mostly run by French or Lebanese businessmen. We divided up the apples to make enough pieces so all the children at the boarding school had a piece. They tasted divine! We stuck together and learned to create something positive out of most circumstances, while we quietly acknowledged each other's dark and scary moments. There was not much else we could do. Children survive but are always affected. Our bodies remember.

I was nine years old, and it was evening. In Africa, it got dark very quickly. Sometimes it seemed so sudden as if the light had been turned off by a switch. Around eight o'clock, we were all in our beds at the boarding school. The lights were off and my roommate, a younger girl suffering from epilepsy, was quietly resting in her bed. I felt responsible to care for her. Suddenly, we heard something prowling outside our window. We heard an ominous growling and did not dare get up and call for help, as our caretakers' room was way down the hallway. Hyenas were outside our window. I found a flashlight and shined it out into the dark and jumped when a hyena flew up towards the window with a terrible growl. It snarled at me as the light beam passed over him. Thankfully, the window was screened, but we were so very scared and felt so vulnerable and helpless. We had regular visits from the hyenas after dark and we were left with a terrible fear that we tucked away and hid. We felt there was no one we could go to for comfort, and I worried about my siblings in their rooms. They probably were very scared too. I was the eldest and I felt responsible for them although there was nothing I could do. I was only nine years old. The feeling of guilt that I could not do what was expected of an older sister, was difficult to carry. The thought of failing them created a feeling of inferiority which I carried through my life. The fact that it was not fair to expect me to carry this burden and it really was the adults who had failed, I only realised and acknowledged fifty years later. That is a long time to carry what is not yours.

At the boarding school, the food was locked up and it was never considered to serve food in addition to regular meals. When playing 'house' outside, we collected flowers, twigs and whatever we could find in nature and pretended that it was food. We drew rooms in the sand, like an architect would draw a house plan on his paper. Fine lines drawn with a stick were the walls between the rooms and the doors would be marked with a rock on each side of the entrance. The 'house in the sand' became our way of dreaming of a home.

During the dry season there was little food to be found out in nature, so imagination had to do and saved our play. And we had lots of imagination as Africa is brimming with it. The children who lived with their parents in this missionary compound were privileged. They had good food in their homes like peanuts, fruit and biscuits and juice. Still, we who did not have anything often, had the most fun. We made fun of everything and laughed. We laughed because from our perspective the others did not understand how tragic the situation was, and we laughed because we were laughing, and the others were not having as much fun as we did. It just was crazy hilarious. Africa taught me to laugh. I had sunshine inside, and it gave me strength.

I remember how the laughter from the African women would fill the air and carry across the village. They also laughed through tragedy and sorrow. They joked around and made fun of the self-importance of the men sitting in the shade under the trees, listening to their radios. A radio was a status symbol at the time. The men seemed to be doing truly little but were still the king on the hill. The women tended the vegetable gardens, carried water home from kilometres away while also carrying their babies on their backs. In the evening after a long day of work they cooked the meals and served the men. The women laughed loudly with a bond of sisterhood. They knew they were carrying Africa and moving things ahead and still today they are a major force in bringing about progress and change. In many cases, they are taking back their power and are healing their past. Humour is important to the Africans. It helps them keep their dignity under humiliating circumstances. Some says humor is holy. I understood and related to that in Africa but forgot it when I moved to Norway. Norwegians did not understand, and I felt hopeless to try to explain.

I must admit not every experience could be handled through humour. Sometimes, it simply just hurts. The fact that children protect their parents is common knowledge. We did this also. We didn't want to bring bad news when we finally could spend time with them during our vacations. Therefore, this sad news was never shared as we simply wanted to enjoy the time at home with our family to the fullest. Our time at home was always full of play, explorations in nature, and a lot of good food. We just did not want to think about our time at the boarding school.

Mum was a good seamstress. She sewed all the clothes we needed when we were home on vacation. After each vacation, we returned to school with new clothes and shoes. We were so proud of our dresses, but very quickly outgrew the shoes. They ended up in the closet while we ran around barefoot. No one cared. One day, we were to celebrate a wedding. A young Norwegian couple was getting married, and it was a big event. It was the first time we had been to a wedding. I did not have shoes that fit and felt very ashamed of the fact. Mum and Dad were so far away, they could have been on the other side of the globe as far as I was concerned. There was nothing I could do about the problem but to mention it to our caretaker, an elder lady.

The newly arrived young missionary couple was immensely popular with the kids because they seemed to care. They made sure to have a special party just for us with games, singing and lots of wonderful food. The only snag was that the caretaker at the boarding school had solved my shoe problem by lending me one of her own high-heeled shoes. I could not really play in those and felt terribly embarrassed, so I finally just snuck home in the dark, leaving the party. It was deeply disappointing. There was nothing I could do about it, so I just stayed quiet and tucked the whole incident away deep inside of me. But my body reminded me of the story 45 years later when it suddenly broke out with severe psoriasis in my hands and under my feet. Our body does not let us forget anything. Not until we heal the emotional wound that was the source of it.

There was little room for personal concerns at the boarding school. I was much taller and thinner than the rest of the children. Maybe I had high metabolism, I do not know, but in any case, the meals were not adequate to meet my needs. I was always hungry and was ashamed of this. It was a real sore spot for me, and a button that some would unknowingly push. I did not talk much as a child, so this issue became my secret pain. Many a time, I was saved by the fruit I found on the trees during the rainy season, and I very much enjoyed the large and juicy mangos. But during the six months of dry season, I had a problem. There was no fruit to be found and I carried the sensation of constant hunger way into adulthood. I still have a somewhat problematic relationship with food. To this day, 60 years later, I always make sure people around me are fed well. It is a way of healing the hungry child within me, I guess.

A few times a year, we stayed with other missionaries to give our caretaker a little time off. It seemed quite random where we were placed. Sometimes we were sent two by two. This was a comfort to us, but it did not happen very often. One weekend, I ended up with a couple I did not know very well. As I was so shy, I missed important information about meals, and I missed many. I went hungry, and they did not think to do anything about it. That day, I went home with a friend of mine. She just needed a sandwich, she said. As she stood there buttering a newly baked piece of bread, I couldn't keep the tears back. They ran down my cheeks. The experience was so hurtful, and I felt so ashamed that I don't remember if she gave me a piece of bread or not, nor if I managed to hide my tears. I just know that today I really feel for children who go hungry. They say that one develops empathy through experience.

As a child in Africa, I enjoyed an unlimited imagination and a boundless inspiration from my surroundings. It set colour to my everyday activities. The Africans told me if I would shout out 'kumare, kumare' to the white stork flying overhead, I would get more of these cool white spots on my fingernails. In

Norway, I was later told this happened because of lack of calcium in the diet. I suppose our imagination can give us more joy than the facts!

I was a good runner and I ran and jumped over shrubs and big boulders with joyous abandon, like a graceful gazelle I told myself. I was in touch with my body and enjoyed it. At night, I would dream I flew way up across the sky looking down on beautiful scenery, away from threats and danger. Sometimes, I had to fly to escape something scary and at other times I was simply flying to enjoy the feeling of freedom and the gorgeous landscape. I was very much a part of 'all that is,' the source of life. I found great comfort in trusting and believing in this source. Somehow, I knew I was not all alone in this Universe.

A childhood memory illustrates how close I was to my authentic spiritual self, my soul. I was a spiritually awake child. This time, we were back home on holiday. I was twelve years old. It was six in the morning and the rooster had already awakened everyone in the small village called Mbe, located in the Duru valley in northern Cameroon. My dad had promised to wake me so I could join him for a morning devotion at the church. I was deeply grateful and happy to be with him that morning. The church was a small and very simple whitewashed mud building with a mud floor and mud benches. Rays of sunlight shone on the small congregation of six or seven people who had prioritised taking a quiet moment before starting the business of the day. I enjoyed every second of this moment. A magical energy of complete devotion was resting on this small group of people on their knees in prayer. This spiritual space moved me deeply. It spoke to the part of me that allowed me to dream of things that seemed beyond me – the part that could lift me out of painful and sad things into a safe and peaceful place. This space within was to become my comfort and saving grace through all of life's varying experiences from then on. My attraction to Spirit was inspired and affirmed here in the darkest of Africa.

While at home during vacation, we enjoyed good food and played joyfully in a safe environment. Sometimes we went on exciting outings or joined Dad when he went hunting. Dad hunted for our food regularly and when we occasionally were invited along, he would wake us up around five in the morning. We had to get to the hunting grounds before it got too hot. We brought along food and drink because we would not be back home before the evening. It was all extremely exciting. Dad brought along a couple of African hunters and they carried their bows and arrows while my dad brought along his hunting rifle. The Africans taught us how to read and understand nature and learn to spot which animals had been there and at what time. They could read everything around them both in nature and in the air. They were good at 'reading the signs'. Africa taught me this.

I still remember one memory from such an outing very well. I heard alarming sounds right in front of me in the tall grass and stopped, standing there without moving as I had been taught. I looked around to see where the others were, but the grass was too tall. I could not signal to them what was happening. After what seemed like an eternity a large, dark wild boar suddenly jumped out of the grass and disappear with an angry grunt. I realised it had been just a few feet away from me. He probably understood I was not about to do him harm, so he decided to get away rather than attack. I was shaken but also felt I must carry some protection with me, because I realized the danger I had been in. I wonder if this experience taught me to not let the fear overwhelm me. Even as a child I had this gift of believing in the unseen "help".

Dad asked the African hunter to chase the boar, but it got away. They are a delicacy. Wild African boar has big hog-teeth and is known to be a dangerous animal. Some say they are more dangerous than lions because they are more aggressive and therefore attack more frequently. Dad was a good hunter, but it became clear that he hardly ever caught any game when we were tagging along. Most likely because of the noise and commotion, but he still brought us along for the experience. I am lucky my father was not taking choices out of fear. We were gifted with an adventure, caring and playful father.

Growing up in Africa is what has made me interested in 'invisible language' and 'reading signs'. The Africans were so good at reading their surroundings, the vegetation, air currents and smells. They would read body language and be led by signs and symbols. They would express themselves in colourful pictures and imagery words. Many years later as an adult I struck up a conversation with a well-known Norwegian actor, and she commented on the fact that I used imaginary-words when talking. I was truly a child of Africa and had adopted the notion that everything around me is alive. This is how the Africa I grew up in functioned and this is how I was shaped.

Everything was expressed as colourful, creative and lavish. That was also expressed by the tradition of the women who tattooed their bodies and faces. They made cuts in their skin and put ashes in the cut which would close and heal. The scars showed signs, codes and symbols. Some were incredibly young when their parents tattooed them with the symbols, which they believed indicated their child's character or life purpose.

Our dear African nanny, Tobi Pauline, was a big, strong, kind and beautiful woman. I was not even one year old when she joined our family. Despite her extremely dramatic life Tobi often laughed. She laughed and joked around while she carried one of us on her back and another on her hip when we were too tired to walk.

Tobi also had tattoos, both on her face and stomach. I had no idea what these tattoos meant until much later when I started to study the language of symbols. I remember Tobi having small, narrow lines indicating steps from the root of her nose and up across her forehead.

Symbolically this indicates a consciousness progression leading to 'awakening,'—the road to heaven—as some Christians would express it. On both sides of her mouth she had lines that looked like a cat's whiskers, indicating her sensitivity. It was most likely a gift that she received at birth and her mother knew it because she had 'read it in the stars.' On her tummy around the navel she had a big sun beaming out in a large circle. This is a known symbol for solar plexus, the centre for self-esteem and strength. Tobi reflected great strength and her energy was shining bright. Strangely this collective old and known symbol has found its way deep into the African savannas, long before they could read or had any contacts with the white man.

Tobi had holes in her nose and earlobes where she placed colourful beads. I admired her tremendously and wanted to pierce my ears and nose just like she did. In my view Tobi was my sun, warming me, nourishing and supporting me.

Tobi had been a slave in the household of the village chief and had been terribly abused, but she had managed to escape to the mission station. She lived there with her husband, Batalimi, who helped us wash our clothes. One day he threatened Tobi, nearly taking her life. This was another side of Batalimi. He was imprisoned and later expelled to Congo, his native country. Life certainly could be rough in Africa.

While Tobi lived with us, she was again abducted by the village chief, who believed she was his property, and my dad had to get her back. He took a great risk in doing so, but that was my dad. On a dark night he took his car and went with a couple of black men to the castle of the village chief to kidnap Tobi back. They found her lying in a corner of a dark room, beaten up and scared. As they carried her quickly out, they had to run for their lives as the chife's men were chasing them. But they escaped. No one could stop my father if he had decided to get something done. He loved people and the battle to end slavery in Cameroon was close to his heart. The force of his heart was big, and I know the energy of Africa inspired him to grow strong. Africa does that.

I was thirteen years old and was going to visit my African girlfriend who lived not far from the powerful chief in Ngaoundere. I was always a little worried to come close to this area of town. It reminded me of Tobi's abduction years earlier, but still it was important to visit my newly married girlfriend. She was also thirteen years old and had just recently been given away in marriage. "Ga fara wå!" I shouted, meaning 'Here I am!' before entering the inner courtyard where the lady of the house was sitting. We embraced each other, and I congratulated her. Then we exchanged gifts. Although we didn't own much, we certainly didn't feel poor. She gave me some thin colourful bracelets made from plastic and I was over the moon. I gave her some colourful glossy pictures. That is all I had to give. Then we sat down to enjoy a shared meal. We ate with our hands from the same dish, laughed and talked about everything young girls are interested in.

My friend found herself confined and restricted. Most likely she did not agree with the match. This whole encounter made a deep impression on me. I think I also feared such a possibility in my distant future. Strangely, at that time I had the idea that I would not like to be married to anybody called John. But somehow, I thought I would not have any choice in this matter, just as my African friend was experiencing.

I knew so little about the power of choices because I had not learned my own will was important. Later I was to learn a lot about this in Norway. Life was to present me with big lessons, and at 23 years old I married John.

The emotional power the Africans show is expressed clearly, both through their fear and joy. Their joy is voiced big and obvious and so is their sorrow. I think no one can suffer and mourn like they do, while on the other hand no one can laugh as loud and abundant as they can. They openly express their strengths and weaknesses. I learned how to laugh loudly, and cry openly and deeply like them. This was the emotional expressions, which to me were healthy and honest. But it did not really seem Norwegians thought the same. It seemed to be too much. Africa taught me the strength of this healthy, sensitive and boldly naked honesty.

To be open is the worst enemy to shame and self-loathing.

– Alberto Villoldo

The shaman (the person who sees and travels between levels of worlds and heals) finds strength in transparency. If you live in harmony with the energies of nature it will protect you. If you have nothing to hide you also have nothing to fear. Only then you are incredibly strong, safe and perceptive.

I was fifteen years old when I had to leave this world of magic and truth. I had to say goodbye to all my African and white friends. I also said goodbye to the nature, the grass, plants and trees in my last few days in Africa. Something told me I would never return to this place. I was in deep mourning as I said goodbye to everything around me that I loved so much. We also had to say goodbye to our second mum Tobi. She begged on her knees to come along to Norway because we were her children. She taught us to walk and talk and was just as much a part of us as a mother. "No, we can't do that," Mum and Dad said.

"Well, then you might as well take out my eyes!" she cried. To be separated from her, created deep wounds in me. It is hard to talk about her without tears welling up even 50 years later. This is also a pain within me that I had to release as I am also proud to have learned to know this power of love and light…She is truly a part of me.

So, I left the playful, intuitive, vulnerable, proud and magical domain where I had experienced such deep sorrow and pain, but also real and strong joy and unrestrained laughter. I had experienced exciting adventures and met such colourful people. *Where the light is brightest the shadow is also darkest.* This is how I experienced Africa – and what I hold in my heart.

Chapter 4
Norway and the Mental Mind

There is a thought in your mind right now. The longer you hold on to it, the more you dwell upon it, the more life you give to that thought. Give it enough life, and it will become real. So, make sure the thought is indeed a great one.

— Ralph Marston

The life of contrasts was really giving me big lessons. Now, Norway was to be my new world. I seemingly needed it all for my growth. An entirely different part of me was to awaken and expand here, but it brought huge growing pains.

One of the first things I experienced, when moving to Norway as a 15-year-old girl, was breaking my right ankle while skiing. It was a nasty break and a strange reflection of how I felt when moving to Norway. I truly felt I lost my balance in life. The connection with a safe foundation was broken. No more play, jumping high and taking airy leaps. I found the place I was standing cold, slippery and dark. Everything seemed baffling and unsafe.

I had arrived in a country where the sober, rational, safe and responsible reigned. Life could not have offered me greater contrast but also the greatest opportunities for growth.

Although, I was Norwegian by nationality, I became a 'white immigrant.' I felt no one understood me, and I did not understand them either. I had landed in a foreign culture with many baffling values. As a Norwegian teenager, many expected me to understand the social codes of my surroundings, and I became painfully aware I had little understanding of these cultural cues. My peers mocked me, and for a long time I could not understand why. I could not understand what I was not understanding! It took quite a while before I was aware of the strange and powerful concept of fashion. I really did not see the point. The music entering the scene in Norway at the time, like the Beatles, was foreign to me. I had been brought up in 'the bush' with little knowledge of European culture. Everything seemed strange.

I also struggled with the Norwegian language, which my teachers did not understand, and it made school a challenge. The consequence was I did not talk much. It took several years before I could comfortably express myself in Norwegian. Estranged in this way, I learned how it felt to be 'different.'

My family came to Norway during winter and had to put on so much clothing it was difficult to move! The boots were stiff and heavy, but very necessary on icy roads, we soon discovered. We found it incredible that people walked on ice, and not only that, but it was also dark midday during winter. We truly had landed in a strange place.

My first encounter with the Norwegian summer was not genuinely nice either. I innocently took a stroll in the woods close to a lake where families were enjoying the short season of warm and sunny weather. We were told it was very safe to take nature walks here. On this first stroll in nature, I noticed a man dressed in a long overcoat standing behind some trees and he started following me. It seemed a bit scary and strange. Suddenly, he jumped in front of me and flashed his naked body. Feeling startled and violated I ran home. I had never experienced anything like this, ever. Growing up in the African bush with supposed 'primitive natives' and their natural nakedness, I had never been scared like this. The Norwegian forest without snakes and wild animals seemed far more foreboding and threatening to me than anything in Africa, after this experience.

Forty years passed before I again ventured out alone in Norwegian nature. Fear had taken hold of me. The seeming unnaturalness of the event scared me and severed my relationship with Norwegian nature. I was so disappointed. Still, everything has at least two sides. Later, I was to receive wonderful gifts and deep pervasive lessons in this country. I was to awaken, become aware and find my strength here. *I grew from a child into a conscious adult.* I was pushed into the edges of what I could endure. No more playing and laughing. I had left the sunshine of Africa in my past, and now this northern country was taking me deep down into the darkest corner within myself. It had a lot to teach me, and mirror for me.

Like the strong and solid houses that are natural to Norwegian culture, our Nordic bodies are also big, strong and tall. As creative beings, we all unconsciously express what we carry within. Our past as warriors is embedded deep in our psyche, a part of our DNA. With this great power follows a great responsibility also to be gentle and humble, and to find the balance is not always easy. It seems a contradiction that Alfred Nobel decided the peace prize was to be handed out in this country, considering our past as war loving Vikings. Norway is currently a large exporter of weapons although we are a small country.

We like to claim to be the world's best in several arenas. I am sure there is some good in having a healthy competitive spirit but arriving here as an outsider, I experienced many people as self-righteous, condemning others who did not meet the Norwegian standard. Norwegians have a strange notion that our society has a good understanding of most things, and we easily forget our civilisation is built on knowledge and wisdom from all around the world.

My first memory of this strange hypocrisy was a sad one. I was sixteen and walking to school when I saw a rough-looking drunk Norwegian threatening a dark man. I noticed that he was African, sober and well-dressed. Still, this shabby Norwegian seemed to feel superior. He was cursing and swearing and telling this poor man to return to where he came from. The African stayed calm. He understood. I hurried on and felt a terrible lump growing in my throat and tears started flowing. *This is how 'my people' are treated here,* I thought, and for a moment I was thankful that Tobi had not joined us.

Many years have passed since then, but I still encounter the same attitude at times. I was only a child in Africa when the thought first struck me that 'one day the Africans will say enough is enough and arise – and I feel sorry for the whites then.' Even as a young girl it was hard for me to fathom that grownup people do not understand that one day everything can change, and they may have to take responsibility for what they have said and done to Africans.

I did not always know how to approach the contrasts I experienced in Norway. *The law of Jante*, 'Don't think you are better than others,' is a saying embedded in the Norwegian psyche. This confused me when I experienced the contradictory expectations when Norwegians also seemed to expect you to become a 'world champion' in everything. What to believe, choose or dare to become was unclear to me. Life was giving me a lot to digest and process.

I had always excelled in drawing but when I turned eighteen, my dad suggested I should try to become a nurse. He knew I had dreams and aspirations along the lines of art, but he was probably concerned about how I would support myself as an artist. I felt a strong and sudden resistance in my body when I heard the suggestion of becoming a nurse. I pulled myself together and managed to clearly say, "No." I had never learned it was okay to disagree with authorities, and I did not say 'no' often, but at that point I felt intuitively my life was threatened. Sometimes life gives you a shove. I realised I had to decide before others would choose for me.

One of my biggest lessons was seemingly to say 'No' and set my own boundaries. This was just the first time I was to be tested, and after that I was given frequent tests of this throughout my life. This time, I chose to listen to my heart and joined art school in Trondheim, studying sculpting. People in this northern part of Norway were more easy-going and this suited me well. I really needed and appreciated this experience to adjust my strained relationship to my new home country. I felt welcomed here, and I knew I was at the right place at the right time.

Synchronistic events confirmed my choice, and everything miraculously fell into place.

As I look back on this time in my life, I can see I listen to my heart and the guidance I received. Still a few more decades passed before I had the courage to fully trust and listen to my heart. I had to take my lessons.

My teacher at the art school in Trondheim, Karl Johan Flaathe, 'adopted' me and became a cherished support and guide. He consistently offered me to phone home from his office. Maybe he thought I was a bit young to live away from home and might yearn to hear news from my family. Little did he know I was accustomed to being away from home and taking care of myself. Still, I was touched by the loving care which I had not experienced before. In this environment, I was welcomed and accepted unconditionally. In the artist community, I realised warmth and kindness can be experienced in Norway. Being different was okay here, and my colourful ways looked upon as an advantage. I started to blossom. Good things were coming my way, but the heaviest part of my lessons was looming in the future and yet to come. My journey had just started.

My life was quite spartan the first little while in Trondheim. I had little money, so I ate poorly. I was not estranged to feelings of hunger, so I told myself to simply accept it. But the Universe wanted to teach me; *I did not have to always expect the worst.*

One afternoon, as we were taking a coffee break at school, Lise, a younger student in our class asked me if I would consider living with her and her family. They had a big house and she would appreciate the company, she said. That day I had a slight fever and realised it could be because of the cold little place I was renting. Lise had also noticed I would do my morning toiletry at school because I did not have access to a bathroom where I lived. Besides this, Lise knew nothing of my disastrous economic situation. I kept that to myself. A bit bewildered, I said yes to her generous offer. She even helped me to move. Life had sent me an angel. The first of many to come.

I found myself living in style and needed to assure that Lise's parents had really agreed to this. Lise's mother replied they were simply very thankful Lise did not have to be alone in the big house while they were at work. Both parents were head physicians and terribly busy.

The next morning, Lise woke me up telling me the nice big, heated bathroom was available. This luxury made me smile as I took my morning shower. I was then invited to breakfast prepared by the maid. Eggs and bacon were something I had only heard rich people having for breakfast. I felt I was living a dream. What a contrasting experience to the situation I just had moved from! Life was playing with me.

After breakfast, Lise dropped me off at the art school before driving off to the university where she was studying. She only joined the art-class few nights a week. At lunchtime, she picked me up in her car and drove home where the maid had lunch ready. Then I was dropped off at school again. I enjoyed every day. This was almost too good to be true. A few weeks went by before I asked to have a little talk with Lise's mum. As I offered to pay the rent she smiled and said she did not need my money! "Just the fact that you add joy to Lise's life is enough for me," she said. I felt deeply welcome and supported. This was a wonderful experience.

I had left Oslo to study art. I moved to Trondheim without a network or money and simply trusting I was doing the right thing. I had followed my heart and taken the leap and was now carried along by the current. I was lifted by a wave of love. Somehow, I needed this experience to strengthen my trust in humankind before the next chapter of my life was to unfold.

While in Trondheim, I started seriously considering becoming a nun and living in a monastery where I could still do art. One day, a group of nuns arrived from a monastery in Stuttgart, Germany. They did extensive charity work but also had artists working in their monastery. Their presence awakened a vague memory from childhood in Africa. I was 13 years old and at home on a vacation in our village in the valley of Duru, when a couple from Stuttgart travelling through this part of Africa arrived in our village late one evening. Mum prepared them some warm soup for supper, before they retired for the night. I remembered the excitement I felt when strange people on their adventures come by. They always made an unforgettable impression with their travel-stories shared at our table. For a young girl who knew truly little about the big world outside of the village, it opened my mind to an exciting 'something' for the future. The name Stuttgart stuck with me, and many years later I was now hearing it again. The synchronicities were unavoidably interesting.

After joining a big meeting, where the nuns presented their order and monastery, I was convinced. I wanted to do this. But before I was able to act on this decision, I met John, the man who I was to have my three wonderful children with. Meeting him turned all my plans upside down.

In hindsight, I have had mixed feelings regarding what this meeting with the nuns from Stuttgart was to teach me. As a small girl, I would entertain myself with dreams about the 'paradise' I was going to build one day. Maybe I unconsciously thought that this life in the monastery could be the alternative or substitute for my childhood dream? Later I understood, it also could have been an unconscious desire to escape from my lessons and a difficult reality in Norway. We do not easily escape from our tasks, teachings or mission!

I was twenty-two years old when I met John. We met in Trondheim and one year later, we were married in Oslo. This marriage was to give me both great gifts as well as great pain. I was to grow to be more aware and mindful. I learned it is not by escaping the difficulties, but rather by facing them that I grow in strength. I was to be strengthened for the rest of my life-journey.

Norway was really a blessing in disguise.

Chapter 5
Dream and Pray

When we answer the call of our heart, we help awaken the heart of the world.
– Marianne Williamson

I am thankful that I saved my journals and now I can see the advantage of doing so. I was not sure they would be of much use when I wrote them, but somehow, I felt it was important to take care of them. I am gaining perspective of my experiences through the journals and am grateful for the memories they evoke, *not as a source of pain but rather jewel of experiences.*

Now, at 58 years old and feeling free, I was sitting in Bandon bravely taking all my notes out to revisit my life. I wanted to get the perspective of it all and to see the bigger picture. I recognised some special gifts that really had supported me well throughout my childhood and later through adulthood, which was the power of prayer and of dreams.

As a child, I learned to turn to prayer for comfort, and as an adult I once again turned to prayer. It helped me to feel I was not alone in this Universe. The life I was living as an adult and a newly married woman, led me through big emotional storms. It was helpful to believe in something greater than myself, as I did when I was a child. I had to believe I was not 'just left and forgotten' here. At the same time, I also grew more conscious about my dreams. I understood they were part of the help I received from universe.

When we feel unbearable pain that is when we look for answers. The dreams, the prayer and meditation were all tools to help me throughout my journey of healing. I learned the language of this hidden Universe. It helped me to awake and to take responsibility of my experiences. My dreams came to be very important to unlock the hidden and finding the source of my pain. The signs and symbols that were given to me throughout my inner journey were the shining lights I needed at every corner on the long and winding road.

About dream.

Dreams are letters from the unconscious. To not take the time to process a dream is like not opening an important letter to us. I learned that making the effort to open and 'read' the dreams gave me exercises and experiences in 'reading' everything I face during the day.

One day I could not find my glasses. I really liked those glasses and whispered a prayer asking for help to find them. That night I had a dream (Chapter 5: Dream nr 4: Flying high above) where I found my glasses behind the bookshelf. When I woke up, I knew they could not be there. I still checked, and as expected did not find them there. Then, the thought dawned on me that maybe I needed to read the books on the shelf. Maybe they would give me the needed insight to something? I started reading all the self-help books I had in the shelfs and bought more. I studied everything I could find regarding interpreting symbols and dreams. I joined workshops on healing and meditation to find some answers. This newfound knowledge became my 'glasses' showing me a new and richer life. I learned to see beyond the physical reality and discovered an even bigger inner world. This new knowledge was awakening me from a life where I did not think I had choices. I learned everything starts in the mind. I had been blind and now I was slowly awaking.

Wishful thinking or daydreaming was often something I turned to in difficult circumstances when I needed sanctuary or a substitute for something I did not have. Thank goodness for daydreams. The dream I had as a child was to create a paradise. This place, where everything was beautiful and safe, was surely born from the loneliness, insecurity and pain I felt because of being separated from my parents and siblings. As a child you do not often reflect on the possibility if your dream will become reality or not. It does not seem so important. Rather it is a sanctuary where you can rest in the hope.

A distinguished African once said in an interview, "You can take a mother from a child, or remove the father, you can take everything of value and the child will still survive. But if you rob him of hope, the spark of life will die!" The spark of life is replenished by hope. Our dreams carry this spark of life originating in 'Source'. American Indians call this 'Source' the 'Great Spirit' that is that 'Force' living in and embraces everything. Great Spirit is the Source of our Hopes.

Don Miguel Ruiz, author and physician from Mexico, became an enthusiastic conveyor of his native shamanic heritage, the Toltec teachings. He describes dreams as an important part of life. 'Dream is Mind's main function, and mind dreams around the clock. It dreams when the brain is awake and when it is asleep. The difference is that when we are awake, we have a material world around us that causes us to perceive things linearly. When we are asleep, we no longer have such frameworks, and the dream tends to change all the time.'

In my dreams, I am free from the limitations of my body. As a child in Africa I often had dreams where I could fly. I remember I could simply decide if I wanted to fly and then just lifted off. It was all so natural and normal but required complete focus and trust. I often dreamt I could levitate when and wherever I wanted. Now, as an adult, I recognised I did not dare to trust this ability anymore. I had become more mental with time and thoughts weigh you down.

I was still married when I had a dream (Chapter 5: Dream nr 4: Flying high above) where I was flying high above a beautiful lush and green landscape. I was strong and free to go wherever I wanted and enjoyed it immensely. Suddenly I became insecure and feared I would not be able to stay up in the air. I was pulled down. The fear robbed me of the ability to fly. The *dream* told me I was allowing worries and fear-based thoughts to overpower me. They sneak up on me like uninvited guests. I later learned those fear-based thoughts can only enter if I allow them to.

"Knowledge gives buoyant for the wings of intuition," I heard a well-known Israeli musician say on the radio one day. The root of the word 'knowledge' is to know what you feel! I had to learn to listen to the feelings of my heart. My heart knows what part of me is ready to fly and it chooses only what is best for me. I had to listen and see through the windows of my soul. 'Dreams are the window to your soul. The real world is within,' Native American Indians say and believe our life is a dream we have created. We have dreamt our conflicts and sorrows into existence because we have allowed fear-based thoughts to create them. But as we feed our thoughts and wishes with visions of a better world, we will through time also dream this into existence. The true paradise we dream of is 'heaven in our hearts'.

Native Indians think our life, what we call our reality, is an illusion and the real life is without fear or pain. The life we are living is therefore simply an experience, an illusion created for learning, as we return to our real selves, our real world or paradise within our Eden.

Throughout my journey I learned we are light, but do not have the courage to believe so. We are creators, but do not take responsibility for what we have created. Our lives are all about waking up to the reality we have inside. I learned that my goal was to become a 'master dreamer', one who consciously creates the reality where all are honouring and serving the Oneness. If I chose to believe in this 'paradise dream' I got stigmatised as an unrealistic dreamer, one who cannot be trusted. In other cultures, to be a dreamer is a badge of honour. The dreams carry visions and intention that help create a new world. I find it strange to choose the 'Vision' of nightmare above the 'Vision' of paradise is more acceptable in our Western culture.

In order to awake from the dream, you need to master the dream.
– Don Miguel Ruiz

I think we would not have the dreams or visions to guide us if we could not access the knowledge to make use of the messages in our dream. The Universe does not waste its resources. Just as we have used parables throughout times to convey new and difficult messages, the subconscious uses dream-symbols to convey knowledge that is otherwise not available to us.

The founder of the Mandala centre in Oslo, Norway, Benedicte This, writes in her book 'Regnbuetreet' (the Rainbow tree), Symbols are God's hidden language found in every living thing. The whole universe is co-working with my soul in its attempt to awake me to be conscious. That is awe-inspiring. When I set out to interpret a dream but feel I do not know enough to do so, I just allow my curiousness to guide me in a playful way. Some shamanistic traditions say we should meet the dream as a reality we are trying to recognise. You can bring out specific elements, persons or situations in the dream and talk to them and ask them what it is trying to tell you.

The dreams are personal, but sometimes we get too close to the picture. To share the dream with others is a great way to look at it from a new angle. My personal interpretation is important, but I might often avoid seeing something simply because I do not want to or are not ready to see it. It can therefore be a great help to get someone else's perspective. The dreams can also have several layers. It may be personal but also speak to the collective, or reflect collective events, since we are a part of it all.

Another way to do dream interpretation is to play with words, pictures and affirmations. The themes that are repeated regularly often show the deepest and most difficult patterns. Nightmares are like big headlines in the newspaper. It is an unprocessed emotion that has struggled for a long time to be heard and therefore must revert to using bold headlines. This emotion will not let go before I have opened to listen.

To connect with my dreams, I must write them down every morning as accurately as I remember them, regardless of how few specifics I remember. I also jot down the day and date I had the dream. In this way, I can more easily spot any patterns that might appear over time. I receive insights into the answers and finally recognise the patterns and message. The dream I have in the night is from a source that is not manipulated or controlled by my fearful ego. It is a pure channel between my higher self and my mind, between heaven and earth. My dreams are the rainbow bridge.

About praying.

When I find the dream too difficult to understand or inaccessible, I pray. 'Prayer is a phone call to God' I read. It requires childlike faith to get connected. Unconditional faith is the key to magical wonders. Mum and Dad often tested 'the word of God'. Ask and you shall receive, it is written. They accepted this literally and in full faith. For missionaries with a small salary and many children the transition to Norway was not easy to handle. Everything costs more here.

One day, right after our return to Norway, the whole family were gathered at the breakfast table. Dad said thanks for the food and closed the prayer by saying, "We have now eaten all the food we have, so let's pray for the money to cover the food budget for the rest of the month." Later, in the same day, the money came through a letter from Dad's sister in Canada. This probably sounds like a cliché, but it is nevertheless the truth. Dad always remembered to say thanks. Gratitude is magical and magnetic.

At the time we moved from Africa, it was winter in Norway. We only have summer clothing, and everyone needed something warmer for the cold winter. Mum knew that she did not have enough cash to properly dress all her seven children. She said a quiet prayer and asked for exactly 1000 kroner (about 130 US Dollar). She did not mention this to anyone. That was a lot of money 45 years ago. Two days later, an acquaintance knocked on the door. She said God had given her this nudge to give Mum 1000 kroner.

To listen.

I have also experienced it is just as important to listen to that small voice when it says to give. I was about seventeen when I had the impulse that I had to send thirty kroner to a childhood friend. We did not see each other often and I hardly talked to him. At that time of my life, I was struggling with terrible shyness and had to overcome this to send him the money. Mum had given me fifty kroner. It was a lot of money at the time and I was very thankful. I knew she had been saving for a long time to be able to give me this money. I figured it could have been in thanks for helping her around the house.

So, I decided to follow my inner voice and send this friend thirty kroners. It is not that I felt responsible to take care of him, but I just knew that I should send him this money. A few days later, he wrote back to me. He was so happy for the money and had prayed for that exact amount to join an event. It can be just as miraculous to give as to receive.

The intention behind the prayer is crucial to the outcome. I must admit my intention often can be vague. Maybe I pray to succeed in an endeavour while at the same time fear that it might happen. Or maybe I have an unconscious expectation that it will not happen, even though I would like for it to happen. 'Everything' responded to my thoughts and dreams! I can stand in my own way by being conflicted in my thoughts and feelings.

I realised when I sent out a prayer the answer could return as a challenge. What seemed like a problem could often be the answer to my prayer. I had to leave myself open to the fact the answers did not always come in a way I wanted or expected. There was a lot to learn about this strange interaction with my higher self. I learned I will only attract what I desire if thoughts and feelings are synchronised. In other words, my faith must be so strong that I feel I already have what I wish for. Then the attraction is activated, and as I am connected to the Source who distributes all requests, it replies.

About meditation.

To be able to connect with my higher self I found meditation to be of a great aid. It helped me to bring light onto my hidden intentions or agenda. Meditation is neither prayer nor daydreaming, but a method to calm the restless mind to be able to just listen.

My teacher in meditation and inner journeys was Kathrine Gyldenrose who is a spiritual guide, a healer and an esoteric teacher in Norway. A defining idea in esoteric teachings is that 'we are all one'. Everything is alive, and we can therefore communicate with everything on every level. I loved it. I was taught by Kathrine to calm my mind thoroughly by following the breath and as I released, I was filled with a quiet calm. I learned to listen to my inner voice, and at the same time I got access to my inner world. Kathrine taught me to trust all the signs and symbols that appeared during these inner travels. When my mind is emptied, it gets quiet enough to receive answers from my higher self or the Source.

The meditation technique I am using is quite simple. I just breathe deeply and let go of all tension in the body as I breathe out. Each time on the in-breath, I imagine a beautiful light above my head that soars into me and fills me up as I also am enveloped with warmth and security. Little by little, I am completely enveloped in this power. In this safe and quiet space, I can simply rest and heal, or interpret dreams. With this tool I can, in an awakened state, pick up a dream and process what I was not able to face while in the dream. I can finish the dream and consciously change the occurrence. This can result in great healing.

Dream, prayer, and meditation are by and large excluded as gift and tools when the rational mind and material values become dominant in a society. We do carry the knowledge of these gifts deep inside as cell-memories. We must step back to recover what we left behind in our race towards development, welfare and future. It is the only way back to our self.

I had to bring along everything I had learned on my journey when dealing with my pain body. The ego was by far too eager to help me forget what I needed to remember while doing this inner work. The ego did not want change. I had to be persevering, loyal and faithful to my true self in this process. I learned to be grateful for the guidance and support I was given through the gifts of prayer and dreams, signs and symbols. They became my support and guidance on my long and demanding journey to awakening and to heal my pain body.

Chapter 6
The Pain Stories

Words and thoughts are tremendous vibratory force, ever moulding man's body and affairs.

– Florence S. Shinn

To be able to heal my physical and emotional pain, I had to know the source of it. Sitting in Bandon and investing from a distance the pain-story of my life in Africa and Norway, made it a bit easier. The perspective is bigger, and I could get a clearer picture. My ego and its emotional waves were not disturbing the picture as much.

Knowing now I had responsibility for everything I had created was hard to handle and face. I had to investigate what was hiding 'backstage' behind the curtain. What was holding my power imprisoned and hiding my inner sun?

I wrote my dreams down every morning as accurately as I remember them, regardless of how few specifics I remember. I always jot down the day and date I had the dream. In this way, I could more easily spot any patterns that might appear over time. I needed to understand and own what I had created by all my own thoughts. They could be inherited or self-created, but I had to own it all to be able to change anything in my life. I had to dive deep into myself.

I had been married for 23 years and I could no more stay in my marriage. I ended up at a loss, confused and alone with nothing but my three beautiful children. How in the world did I end up here? Where to go next? As I asked dreams appeared with exactly what I needed to see and process. I had a dream (Chapter 6: Dream nr 5: In a large old house) where I was sleeping in a large, old house. It was dark and raining heavily outside. Someone knocked firmly on the old, large and heavy wooden entrance-door at the first floor. I was sleeping deeply in my bed on the second floor. It took a while before I woke up and tumbled down the stairs to the entrance. My mother and father were standing outside in the darkness and rain. Dad was dressed in a long black robe and my mum in a long white one. They were impatient and tired and simply wanted to deliver a package. It was seemingly something especially important, although it was wrapped in modest brown paper. After delivering the package, they left, not saying a word and returned into the rain and dark.

Waking up, I meditated on the dream. In meditation, I know the fear will loosen its grip and I can safely confront what I need to see. My parents came to me in the dream with something they wanted me to 'take a closer look' at. It was a personal gift, something inherited. Over time, I realised this package had the information I needed to guide me in learning to understand who I truly am. They were the gift.

The packaging showed me it really was not anything to brag about. I had a strong impression it was rather the values and the life they had lived that I was asked to take a closer look at. 'Look at us and learn more about yourself', seemed to be the message. The darkness outside seemed to symbolise the sub-consciousness of the collective. The night is also the time of healing.

I interpreted the rain in this dream to be of cleansing the grief and sorrow of our story. The dream showed me to take note of *the contrasts* that my parents represented in their relationship. They both appeared in long robes where the feminine and masculine energy was distributed in a somewhat unorthodox way. Dad was dressed in black robe which symbolises a feminine and creative energy. Mum was dressed in white robe which symbolises a masculine, mental and spiritual quality. Both are a part of me. I was shown I must start using these qualities in my own untraditional way. I need to embrace and balance the opposites or contrasts in my life according to my own heart and free myself from old patterns of behaviour and thinking.

The big, old house represents the body of my heritage. I must find my way out of old habits and inherent addictions that have been passed down through generations in this old family lineage. In the dream, I had been asleep on the second floor. According to the teachings of the East the second level of energy-centre in our body symbolises creativity, desire, pleasure and focus. I had to wake up from my sleep, which in this case symbolises an unconscious life on autopilot. I had to embrace all the gifts in an awakened and conscious way. The gift I received this rainy night is the greatest gift parents can give to their children –

that is themselves. They mirror everything in me. The truth always sets you free, and I was impatient to be set free.

Don M. Ruiz talks about our collective life as a sleep-state, which he describes as a poisonous addiction. He uses the analogy of poison to describe all the negative we are exposed to from birth, through words and attitudes. We have become unconscious and forgotten who we really are, and only believe what we have been told we are.

To be able to change my life and wake up to who I really am, I had to save myself from the collective fog. This included letting go of illusions of limitation and fear-based attitudes, which is part of our collective heritage. This seemed important but near impossible to do. Still, I continued the long and difficult process, taking one step at a time. Once I have found that what I was is not who I am, there is no returning. I was now a seeker of truth.

I was 23 years old when I married, and 23 years later I had to let go. It is strange how we find our lives going in cycles. The years in this marriage became challenging and difficult, but there are also blessings in every experience. In addition to the insight these experiences afforded me my three children. They are the biggest blessings life has given me. They were at this point in my life luckily on their own path of a successful life.

I was on my own now – facing my own truths. When I summed up what I had created during my years of married, I saw the following picture: It had clearly been a crazy race. I was newly married and my beautiful and wise son, Mikal, was one year old when I resumed my studies at art school in Oslo. After four years, I had the Diploma in hand. Mikal was five years old when I was pregnant with my gorgeous daughter June. For economic reasons, I had to work on the weekends at a nursing home for MS patients. When my art-education was completed, I started to work full time at the nursing centre as I also tried to breathe life into my artistic ambitions. At the same time trying to take care of my children. The children's dad was gone lot of the time on his business trips or endless meetings.

I rushed through several years in this manner. At 35, I had my third child, Jan Mathias, a lovely, lively and happy boy. Now, I had three children, but any way, I quickly continued my crazy and hectic life. I even took more responsibility as the representative for the labour committee at my workplace. Somehow, I also was able to make my own art gallery in Oslo, while juggling it all with my night-shift job at the nursing home and my children. Additionally, I, of course, engaged in the local art association and ended up leading it for a while.

I did not see the madness of this lifestyle, but simply felt pulled in every direction. If I was asked to help with anything, 'Yes' was the only reply I had. 'No' was not in my vocabulary. I only slept about four or five hours at night for years. I forgot to breathe and burned the candle at both ends. I was bound to crash at some point.

The last five years of our marriage we lived in a large house where I had a studio many artists could only dream of. I worked hard to participate with exhibitions and promote my art. It was not easy to create when being so stressed with all the other duties I took on. I still managed to join several exhibitions and had a good turnover.

Everyone was happy with me if everything 'paid out'. But it was, of course, unsustainable to keep up with this lifestyle and slowly but surely, I started to lose the spark needed to be creative. Unbeknownst to me, I was about to slip into a deep depression. The foundation was crumbling and again I experienced losing my footing, the way I did when coming to Norway and breaking my ankle. It is strange how things repeat themselves. Life was trying to wake me up, but as a sleepwalker it is not much awareness in our choices.

Around this time, I had a dream (Chapter 6: Dream nr 6: Feeling trapped) where I was flying high up under the ceiling of my big and beautiful art-studio. In the dream, the room was large and beautiful with gorgeous renaissance paintings on the walls and in the ceiling. The floor was a big swimming-pool filled with water. It was thrilling to fly around there but the ceiling stopped me. Suddenly I started to feel trapped and in despair noticed that I was losing altitude. There was nowhere to land and I was afraid I was going to drown in the pool. I woke up confused and unhappy.

In this dream, my studio represents my potential – and my inner workshop. The paintings represent my creative heritage and the ceiling represents the limitations in my life. I was not free to fly. The water showed me, I did not have any safe footing. Water symbolises feelings and creativity which here was found trapped in a pool. In this dream, I see it as a symbol of infinite streams of collected tears. I was afraid of drowning in my own sorrow. I was not safely anchored to anything in myself or in the marriage, and as a result I was not able to create. My heart was not grounded.

I had many dreams throughout my whole marriage where I continually found myself betrayed and humiliated. I still lived in the hope that one day I would receive what I had longed for in our relationship – I just had to be patient, I told myself. I did not realise I allowed myself to get manipulated to the point of continuously suppressing my needs and desires, and I did not realise it had to do with my own choices. It was hard to admit I had the responsibility for my off-the-track life.

The man I was married with was one of the directors in a big institution and was away much of the time. I had mentioned to him several times what I felt about the lack of balance in the responsibility towards the children but was too soft-spoken, obviously. I had never learned that it was okay to speak up regarding my own needs. On the other hand, he never had a problem with helping himself or making himself the priority of our shared resources. I allowed it, basing it on a mistaken kindness. *One day he'll see and meet my needs also,* I thought. I had not understood I was contributing to creating this dysfunctional relationship by not setting boundaries. To always be considerate of his needs became a dangerous and misunderstood attitude which only created more imbalance in our relationship. He was free to use his time, strength and resources on everything but the children and me. This lack of ability to set boundaries for myself eventually caused the breakdown of my life.

While growing up, I never learned to value myself. My voice was not of interest at the boarding school. I learned I was invisible and not important. This was not a good precursor for a good, equal, respectful and loving relationship in the future. With this lack of self-love, I could not see or disclose what my own motivation was behind the choices I made either. As they say, you do not get acknowledged by others unless you acknowledge yourself. This is the law of cause and effect. I was waiting for my husband to change till I finally understood that it was only about my own choices and me. I needed to change my perception about my story and myself.

Turn your scars into stars.

– Dr Robert H. Schuller

It was with painful relief that I, at the age of 45, decided the best thing I could do was to leave the marriage which now represented all my learned dependence, escape mechanisms and denials. I realised I just as well could be honest. I understood it was a big illusion to believe we can keep anything hidden. At one point everything will become visible. Everything you must hide weakens you, I learned.

At this point, I so much wanted to understand everything; who I was and why had I rejected myself so pitilessly? I looked back into my history, to the old ancestral house, to gain understanding regarding the connections and reasons behind all what I had created. Little by little I realised the unconscious memories of rejection in childhood had created a pattern in my life that had been repeating itself.

As a child I compensated for my own wounds by helping others with their loneliness, wounds and feelings. I 'filled' their cups as best as I could, so they would not have to feel rejected. This dulled my own pain momentarily. But it was only a temporary fix, a derailing.

I became dependent on others being well, so I did not have to mirror my own pain.

The memories of rejection had settled in my cells and were strengthened by constant affirmation. As ripples in water, the patterns had repeated themselves and influenced every decision I made into adulthood. Of course, I attracted a man who did not give me much emotionally. It was just a result of my lack of self-love. The law of cause and effect became obvious as I looked back at these choices. Like attracts like. Time gave me perspective and the picture came slowly clearer.

All the emotional pain had manifested itself into physical pains at this point. I had done everything in my power to be loved and accepted in my marriage. I went as far as I was able. Now, the body had to finally use tough measures to stop me. I suddenly had an inflammation in the back and they also detected calcifications in the neck. As the doctor studied the X-rays, he asked if I had ever been in an accident. I had not as far as I knew. "Well, this x-ray shows a neck of a 70-year-old," he said. "It is very calcified."

Not surprised, I heard a little voice inside saying, "You have been carrying a very heavy burden."

The doctor said my joints were too stretched and this explained the inflammation and pain in all joints. "Yes, I've always allowed myself to be stretched further than I really could handle," I responded. My body was reflecting my life. I had to start to listen.

The suffering has a noble purpose, the evolution of consciousness and the burning of the Ego.

— Eckhart Tolle

Moving on. I did not bring much with me when I divorced and moved out of our house. But I was relieved. I had 'saved myself'. People at my work helped me with a flat and I moved in with my two youngest children. My oldest was 22 and already had his own place. Then I continued the hectic pace as if nothing had happened. After only one year, my body and psyche said stop – again. I had moved out of my hurtful marriage but had not invested any time in processing the breakup or 'the wounds' I had contracted throughout these years of marriage as well as those of my upbringing. I was now diagnosed with burnout, depression and fibromyalgia. I was dead tired and looked at the world through a fog when the doctor asked me to take a one-year break. He suggested I should sign up for a course called 'The Wild Woman'. I did not really understand what it was all about but was very touched by the concern and the fact that I was taken seriously. I had not told him much about my personal circumstances, but he read the symptoms and understood.

It is amazing how our psyche manages our lives. Now, at last, my body and spirit allowed me a time-out to replenish my body and mind. This time of admission sent ripples throughout my body from deep inside. In search for answers, I came across information that shook my very foundation and all I had ever believed to be true. 'You Can Heal your Life' by Louise Hay was one of the books I read now. The author brought me to an exciting, although provocative insight into understanding of our own responsibility for our health and lives in general. She had had an almost unbelievably traumatic childhood and adolescence, but she had found a way out of the suffering. Her book inspired me to get a grip on my own life. I was helped to get back on track and gained a greater understanding and practical insight into the metaphysical reasons behind the different physical symptoms I was struggling with.

I 'accidentally' came across more books that presented me with a broader view on human existence. The teaching that I as a human, am part of everything was a liberating, but also scary thought. If everything is connected, it also means that we are all responsible for everything happening in our world. This was at first a hard one to swallow. I then read that everything has its own energy and unique vibration. This made sense to me. I had always been able to sense energy but not really understanding what it was. I also read even feelings have their own energy, a vibration affecting mind and body. This led me to really want to expose and understand my own feelings and the reason of them.

All these mysterious angles to life were now lining up to be seen and understood. "What are you going to do with all these feelings?" the psychologist asked me when I got in touch for counsel and help. I did not really understand what he meant. All I knew was that I was 'very sensitive' and I, for some reason, struggled much more with this sensitivity here in Norway. Is it possible *not* to have all these emotions?

In Africa, the emotions were strong and visible. The sun was shining warmly and intensely, and the violent tropical downpours would also flood my senses. This contrast was mirrored both in the Africans as well as the rest of us growing up there. As a child I was never told to keep back my tears or my outbursts of joy, nor the loud and happy unbridled laughter. But I learned that in Norway this was not acceptable.

Many now acknowledge the gifts of extremely sensitive or emotional people. Thankfully, we are not as quick to judge it as a neurosis currently. As a newly arrived immigrant and sensitive youth, I was told to wipe that 'smile' off my face. I interpreted it as making too much of myself. The African sun shining through obviously provoked my sober Norwegian surroundings.

I was afraid not to be understood and accepted so I decided to hide my Sun. The fact that I had to hide my Sun, my inner joy, showed up to be harming both my body and mind. The Sun I was suppressing was burning inside of me. I tried unconsciously to compensate by 'doing more' and getting as much done as possible. This is how I came to experience a 'burn-out'. To burn inside or having a burnout are the same thing and a mismanagement of energy. Our body is telling us what we need to know, and we must listen. The trouble was I wasn't listening yet.

Realisations.

As a 45-year-old divorced and sick woman, I had to discover what I was not understanding yet and what was blocking me from understanding. The process was demanding. Family and friends can give help and support through the grieving process, but one day you find you have been repeating the same story so often that you must find another solution.

I found journaling to become an important part of the solution for me and a faithful companion. I learned by writing down thoughts and experiences in the journal that it was not so easy to escape and run away from them. This helped to spot patterns in my life, no matter how unpleasant.

I saw I had learned to reject myself for so long that my body received the message as if I did not want to live, so it started shutting down. Mind and body had to be rewired. But it could not be done by simply flipping a switch. There were many layers of self-destructive and hardened thought patterns as well as patterns of behaviour to work through. My body just tried to help by showing me.

Burn-out: I had no energy/fuel left. The engine cuts out when it runs out of oil. I had not taken the time to stop and refuel at any time.

Depression: It was my mind telling me that I had given up and was feeling overwhelmed. It also expresses withheld anger and unreleased power.

Fibromyalgia: is an expression of infected thoughts regarding oneself and life in general. It had now invaded all muscles and joints. Joints symbolise mobility and flexibility of mind or thought, and the muscles support action.

My choices had not been supportive of my true self and my body expressed it in ways it knew how. I had to become aware of what it wanted to tell myself. Regarding my childhood some doctors and psychiatrists also diagnosed me with 'post-traumatic stress syndrome'. In his review of my case, Dr Berthold Grunfeld, a prominent Norwegian psychiatrist (now deceased), clarified that there is not much one can do with these diagnoses but to let them heal with time. So, there wasn't much help to find and I didn't want to start with any medication. I had to find the underlying cause resulting in taking the self-destructive behaviour so far. How could I break this pattern and how could I learn to love myself back to health?

Once more. Time passed, and I now had reached fifty. As I was getting a bit of distance to my marriage of twenty-three years, I started to experience shame about the fact that I had not done something sooner to get away from this humiliating relationship. This feeling would not let go. But I did not understand the seriousness of not dealing with it and therefore jumped on the roundabout once again. I did not want to accept the fact that you really cannot run from your problems. I continued my education as an art teacher and stubbornly threw myself into the maelstrom of everyday life, simply just wanting to feel 'useful' again. I probably had something to prove also, especially to my children, as I understood the whole situation had been taxing for them as well. But I still had not learned the importance of the balancing act between body and mind.

Then of course, it happened again…I had only worked for a short while as an art-teacher before I lost my footing and collapsed – again. I was still too weak to handle pressure and adversity. I had the capability but still not the strength and ability to put my foot down where and when needed. The lack of strength made me feel powerless, insufficient and subservient. It hurt to have to face that I was not coping with the pressures of everyday life. It is not easy to check out from society's expectations and fellowship. You become very vulnerable and alone.

We mirror the society we live in, and I had abused myself, my time and my talents. I was mirroring a society where most choices are made from fear. Fear that a budget will not balance, that a boss will give a scolding or stop a cherished project. It could be fear that workmates will not like me or fear of getting fired. Maybe I force myself to move on despite being wounded, fearing the fact that loved ones are not able to understand my condition. The fear takes many shapes based on unconscious intention.

I had to learn the same lesson over and over before I was willing to admit my limitation and gather the courage to I had to allow time to become my friend, not my enemy.

I found this so hard. Time had been part of the threatening image creating stress in my life. I read somewhere time really is an illusion, simply part of our linear reality. I had believed in a limited universe with little time and the ceiling low, the rooms small and resources limited.

One day, someone was teaching me about an unlimited universe. It felt wonderful and gave so much hope whether it was proven true or not. A friend asked me to join her in a gathering at the University in Oslo where the spiritual leader Sri Sri Ravi Shankar was participating. My body was hurting, and I was not comfortable on the hard seating. As the guru asked us to join in a meditation where he was going to initiate several in the audience who were ready for this, I started to feel very unsettled. I had never participated in anything like this before and how in the world was I to relax and meditate with this excruciating pain in my back? I still wanted to try and closed my eyes while breathing deeply. I turned my attention towards the voice of Sri Sri Ravi Shankar. For a moment, I forgot all about myself and suddenly I was flying way up in the sky! I could not see the earth beneath me, as there were lots of beautiful sparkling clouds in many colours above and beneath me. I flew at a tremendous speed between these colourful bright clouds. In amazement, I enjoyed the freedom and beauty around me and was carried forward at an unimaginable speed. Then abruptly and firmly, I was back in my body and surprised found myself back on the uncomfortable bench.

This was my first experience travelling unrestricted but conscious in a non-physical world and for a short while I was transported out of a painful reality. I told my dad this outlandish experience in the hopes that he could explain to me about the phenomenon. He had both studied and taught religion history for many years. He looked at me quietly for a while and then said that I had probably been astral travelling. Thankful and a bit surprised that my dad knew about this phenomenon, I hid this amazing experience in my heart – as a flickering light deep inside of me. I knew I had received a precious gift and an insight into a big internal universe; a reality without my pain-story and limitations. I was free if I dared to be.

Chapter 7
Role-play

Until you dare to dream a new story, all you will have is the nightmare.

– Alberto Villoldo

To know something is quite different, then to acknowledge – and live it.

I was still holding on to stories which made me feel neither free nor healthy. I was in a process of getting better now but I had to go deeper into what was holding me back. Something was holding a part of me hostage. My body and mind were just starting to express what was not released yet. Time had passed. I did not feel any big development health-wise, although I thought I did what I could do to aid in the healing. The symptoms seemed reluctant and deep-rooted. Could these wounds have been created and supported by the different 'roles' I had taken on throughout life? Had I inherited it? Were those roles disguising the source of the pain? I wondered. I had to reveal who and what they were, and what was their purpose?

I felt lost and so unbelievably vulnerable—as if I were a child without any guidance—except for my dreams. One night, I dreamt (Chapter 7: Dream nr 7: A little girl on the stage) I was watching some children being taught acting on a big stage in an old theatre. The teacher seemed quite stern and authoritarian. It was late evening. One child had not arrived, and another was to take her place. A shy little girl who was standing at a distance admiring the play, was asked to step up and play the part. She did not know the dance and did not understand the choreography and therefore was very anxious, but she still picked up the courage to step up and do it anyway. Suddenly, the ceiling opened showing a high black sky covered with stars. She looked up at the stars and 'read' what she needed to know in the stars. Somehow, she was able to learn what she needed through listening to what the stars showed her. I woke up with a sense of warmth and peace.

The little girl was not particularly pretty or talented, I thought, but she was so cute and brave. I knew this little girl lived inside of me. I understood I would be led by the universe, if I took up the challenge, trusted and participated on the stage of life. The dream wanted me to wake up and to take interest in this brave and clever little girl within me and her dreams. I had to step up on this internal stage to learn to know her and listen to the guidance of the stars and the universe surrounding her. I felt inspired.

Intuition is a spiritual faculty and does not explain, but simply points the way.

– Florence S. Shinn

What roles had I been playing throughout life? In my study I found a character is often an unconscious personality-trait which is played by one of three archetypes: the abuser, the victim and the rescuer. I learned: The abuser (or bully) is the one manipulating and controlling his environment – even if only subtly. The bully can play on people's fear or weakness. The victim is the one who claims that the environment is not paying enough attention to them. They let others make the decisions but then complain about them. The victim thinks that life owes them something. Oddly enough, the victim can quickly become the abuser, manipulating their surroundings through their suffering. The lines can get a little blurry here. The rescuer always thinks that she must help, save or do something for others. They also often step into situations where they have not been invited or where they are not even needed, because they are dependent on being needed. In this case also the role as rescuer can develop to become a manipulative abuser. All the different characters can seamlessly bleed over into each other. I recognised myself in all of them. There was certainly a lot of work to do.

In the book, 'The Four Insights' Alberto Villoldo writes about the challenge we meet when we give up our old characters. It is scary. They had been my safe place and I know I would feel naked without them. The challenge is to acknowledge the power within us without needing to play any of these roles. Alberto Villoldo compares this process with the snake shedding its skin to continue to grow. The snake does not believe it is the old skin. I am not my old story nor the old character that I had been playing out! I can let it go.

Recognising old thought patterns helps me better see whatever no longer serves me. Finally, I had started to unwrap the brown package my parents gave me in that dream (Chapter 6: Dream nr 5: In a large old house) one rainy night. The gift was my parents themselves. I had to investigate their roles and characters to enlighten the emotional mysteries hiding inside me. I was a mystery to myself and needed to dive into those hidden gifts.

We inherit many of our response patterns but are not able to change any of them until we take responsibility for everything we hold on to. I had to study the roles of my parents, as they are the most important role-models I grew up with: My dad was a kind and happy person but had a volatile temper and an authoritarian manner that sometimes scared me as a child. Because of this, I became afraid to accept my own temperament and inner strength. Deep inside, I recognised my power, but I locked it up not to scare people the way I had been scared. I later learned if I am afraid of this power it turns against me. This power would find a corner in my nature where it could hide and every now and then cause me to feel anger, but mostly it became hostage to my fear.

I learned the reason for having a father who reflected this strength, was to teach me to face it and learn to deal with it, not run away or try to hide from it. I could have seen this force as a great gift – if I had only faced and conquered my fear. Dad was impulsive, strong, social, adventurous and with a wonderful great childlike joy. He genuinely loved people and had big visions and dreams. This is wonderful heritage to pass on. But to ignite everything I am into action, I needed to recognise this strength within me. My inner strength was big but not yet acknowledged by me. It was like a sleeping giant – or a gorilla.

Instead of bringing out the power I had in me, I had played the role of the kind and patient 'rescuer.' This became the unconscious role of ego through my whole adolescence. Playing this character gave me some gain in the short term but long term it stopped me from living my own life to the fullest. I still clung to this self-image. I did not see I was robbing myself through this act. The sense of 'responsibility' which legitimised these roles I was playing became a pattern, the DNA permeating my whole old ancestral house. I was struggling with patterns of the co-dependency, of 'being needed.' I studied my ancestral house while at the same time seeking the help of therapists and healers. I wanted to get well and of course I did not think my healing process was going fast enough! A part of me was a tyrannical inner partner.

By and by my therapists concluded I had access to the answers myself. There was somehow some payback for everything I had read and studied. They acknowledged I understood how I ticked well, and I could interpret my dreams better than they could. It seemed to me they could not (or dared not) connect the information between body and spirit the way I did – and gave up working with me. From this point on I had to take all responsibility for my continued growth. This may be what my soul wanted me to do: take responsibility of my life.

The old unconscious idea that I needed 'to hurry' was pushing me forward. The idea of not having enough time for my process was just the fear of not being accepted and successful. I wanted to move on, and once again I thought I was ready to take on new challenges. I joined a workshop about 'Starting your own business.' Now, I wanted to use everything I had learned going through my own process to 'help others', and I was quite sure I was ready to tackle it, strangely enough. How ironic.

I wanted to start a centre for art therapy and spiritual guidance. Many had encouraged me to try this path. I knew I was competent and passionate in teaching and counselling. I had now become an adjunct, specialising in art and had also taken courses studying art therapy. The next step was to look for the right location to fulfil the dream. After a long search, I was about to give up when it dawned on me that I had to stop and allow myself to be guided. I let go of everything I thought, I had to, ought to and should do and popped by an alternative bookstore run by some friends of mine.

There I settled down with a cup of coffee and an interesting book when the door opened and in strode a beautiful young woman. She started up a conversation with the owner of the shop who she obviously knew. I heard her mention she was on her way to a centre in Grønland, an area in the central of Oslo. I knew right away that I had to go there. When I arrived, I was greeted beautifully by the owner Eirik Myrhaug, a known Norwegian shaman. In the first place, he just had in mind to rent out one of the rooms, but when he understood I was interested in a bit bigger place, he surprisingly offered me to take the whole place. I just said yes! How wonderful!

This was just what I hoped for.

The centre became a community for several therapists and healers. We shared the large communal room for meditation groups, seminars and lectures.

The centre grew, and people were thriving. I held courses covering dream interpretation and intuitive painting. I had private consultations upon request and some lecturing assignments and workshops for private and public establishments. My gifts developed and grew stronger according to the challenges I took upon me. I enjoyed being a teacher and guide and received much good feedback. Soon my schedule was fully booked.

Seemingly everything was good…But strangely, something deep within troubled me. Something uncomfortable had been left unattended while I was busy 'helping others'. I had forgot something especially important on my hasty way ahead. Again.

All disease has a mental correspondence, and in order to heal the body one must first heal the soul.

– Florence S. Shinn

I learned our gifts can also become our stumbling blocks. At the same time, what I struggle most with can finally become my strength. I loved to guide and help, but I had to balance this gift with tending my own needs. I had not yet integrated this lesson. I had to learn to take better care of myself. Why was this lesson so difficult for me to learn?

All the pain in my body had been playing up in the background all the time, and now was coming to the fore again. In my attempt to ignore it, it had only grown stronger.

Suddenly, adding on to all the other symptoms, I now developed a severe outbreak of psoriasis inside both of my hands and under both of my feet. It was very painful to walk on gaping wounds and soon I could not use my hands. I could not have received clearer signs. I was not supposed to do anything or go anywhere!

I had thought I could 'will' myself well and had not consulted with my own heart.

'Be gentle with yourself' was the message I got. Oh, so hard. Nobody had taught me that!

I had been wearing too many hats and playing all the roles on the scene! In running the centre, I had not learned how to delegate responsibility nor to set boundaries for myself. So, I was still playing the role of 'saviour and helper' without considering my own needs. To be honest, I was my own 'abuser.' I had not listened to my inner child that knew how to look to the stars and read the signs. I had not listened to my authentic self. It was more difficult than I had thought to change behavioural patterns. I was still dependent on my role-playing, and still 'robbed' myself to 'rescue' others. Once again, I was forced to turn my focus inward. I had to read myself more carefully with more of an open, compassion and caring heart. My body was giving me some tough signals.

The skin symbolises our identity. It protects us and shows our boundaries. It is also the largest organ of our body. My psoriasis showed me how I felt about myself. Not too good and too wounded. The wounds under my feet showed me I was not standing on safe ground within myself yet. I had not found my footing or a good balance before once again taking on new roles and responsibilities. The wounds in the palm of my hands also showed there was not a balance between what I gave and what I received.

And of course, I got a dream (Chapter 7: Dream nr 8: I was warned.) with a clear warning: I was standing high on the tip of a mountain peak and was a bit wobbly on my feet. The wind was blowing fiercely, and I had nothing to hold on to. I tried to keep my balance the best way I knew how, while looking down in terror at the foot of the mountain many hundred feet beneath. There was no safe way to get down. I woke up sensing an intense fear flowing throughout my body.

The dream told me I had climbed up to a place, a pedestal, where I could not see any way out of my debility. I felt like a victim of circumstances although realising that I got myself there. The wind blowing so fiercely symbolised the chaotic thoughts tearing at me. It was expectations and ambitions I and others had placed on me. I was trapped in my own choices!

There was no other way to get down than to let go and allow myself to fall. I had to let go of the centre. To 'let go' was to become one of my hardest lessons and deepest learning.

Yet another round of recognition was needed. The characters I was trapped in were deeply ingrained in the person I thought I was, and my ego was a strong protector of it. I realised if I do not own all my experience, I also do not own the possibility of change. This work takes a close teamwork between heart and mind. I had to find true communication between wish and desire, body and spirit, heart and mind.

I had allowed myself to get manipulated by the expectations. I still had not understood it is a choice to allow myself to be manipulated. The ego expresses itself in the characters I am acting out and gets strengthened every time I allow fear to guide my choices. The ego got a lot out of the characters I identified with and it did not care about the resulting pain. To let go of everything known and let life lead me into the unknown, and what my heart was truly longing for, was risky but necessary. And, of course, it was a big threat to my ego.

We turn to God for help when our foundations are shaken, only to learn that it is God who is shaking them.

– Charles C. West

Now, I was once again led to go inward. I was not to do anything – but simply to be.

I closed my eyes and sat there quietly listening to the chaos and pain inside. Suddenly I 'heard' a big smile and one thought filled my whole being. "It seems that it is only under these circumstances that you see and listen to us!" I realised the challenges and defeats I had chosen in my life were necessary to discover the assistance which is always there, waiting. I was reminded to truly listen, and this required silence.

I had to step out of shoes that no longer fit me and take off hats that were only borrowed. There was only one thing to do: I had to throw in the towel and do like the bear – go in hibernation. I had to be in total silence to be able to meet 'the one who observes,' the one behind thought—the pure light—my true self. The old reality, my 'pain body', had veiled who I really am. I had to blow away the fog before finding my inner dream world – my Avalon.

The cocoon:

I was on my journey exploring my inner self, onto the Yellow Road of the Rainbow Bridge: the road of knowledge and self-awareness. It was time to find a silent place for my heart to rest and restore. It was time for relaxing, processing, releasing and redefining who I am, and of all my gifts.

In this night of the soul, memories and experiences are being processed to finally give me a new encoding. In this inner sanctuary everything is dissolved to be recreated into a new form. Here I prepare for the next cycle of expansion – in line with my Divine Life-plan.

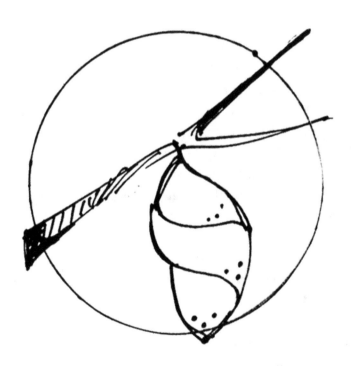

Chapter 8
The Gifts of the Rainbow

And as we let our own light shine, we unconsciously give other people permission to do the same. As we are liberated from our own fear, our presence automatically liberates others.

– Marianne Williamson

If I could not travel out into the world at this point as I was sitting in my living-room, sick and trapped, I could at least take the journey into my inner world. I wanted to understand who Gro really is without the old roles and what was her true-life purpose. The tasks we are given are always in line with our gifts and dreams. I learned I really had access to the knowledge and help needed. I heard my heart whisper, 'Relax, release and receive!' This sounded like a good formula. I had to sit still with no way to escape but to do the self-healing work. I had to only focus on my inner landscape now.

Somehow, I was doing something right my heart told me by giving me an encouraging dream (Chapter 8: Dream nr 9: Rainbow in the lagoon). I was standing in the grass by a beautiful lagoon surrounded by hills and lush vegetation. I noticed light rain and suddenly a magnificent rainbow stretching from land and out into the centre of the lagoon. It started suddenly to rain harder, but I still decided to get out into the water. A strong current made me uneasy, and I heard several people on shore warning me to be careful, but I had made up my mind and struggled my way out to my treasure, in the end of the rainbow.

No one could stop me now.

The dream told me it would be a big challenge and a long journey to reach what I longed for. I was not quite sure what the treasure was about, but I told myself I would understand when I 'arrived'. Now, I simply had to follow the rainbow that is the symbol of the bridge between heaven and earth, spirit and matter! I was inspired to study everything I could about the world of symbols. This was the only way to reap the gifts of my dreams, I had to invest in them! 'Read the signs!' had over time become like a mantra to me.

I read the dream to the best of my ability using the information I had at the time. I had been given time and space to get everything I had learned and achieved through my educations and experiences into use. All the tools I found on my journey and throughout my life, and all the knowledge I had acquired, I now could use to interpret my dreams and signs that universe gave me. In the Bible the rainbow symbolises the promise between God and man to be protected. The rainbow also is a universal symbol of our inner travels – through every level. It has been described as a mystery travel, the seven rays of light, as well as the seven chakra centres in the auric structure. Benedicte. This is a well-known artist, author and spiritual coach in Norway. In her book *Regnbuetreet* (The Rainbow tree), she writes about the rainbow as a symbol of the consciousness ladder and the key to 'all of nature's secrets'. The rainbow gives a guidance towards my gifts within and promises me protection. It shows the way through the process and gives support on my Earthly journey.

Water is the element of creativity, feelings and birth. It cleanses and gives nourishment to new life. The rain, wind and current revealed to me that I would meet both mental and emotional resistance throughout the journey. It would take toil and tears as well as great courage. But I really did not have a choice, because what I wanted to find there in the 'lagoon' was the gifts within me.

The fact that this dream was a peek into the future and what I was going to experience a couple of years later, became another confirmation of the magic of dreaming. We do not have to consider time in dreams and therefore can travel free from the limitations of time and space. The dream can transport us backwards or forwards in time, or even transport us to another dimension or different galaxy. Because of these timeless paradigms, prophecies and predictions are also possible through the dream.

In search for more information and knowledge, I turned to abilities that I already had developed. As an artist I knew the colour contrast bring out the form in the picture, but even more important to the impression of the form are the contrasts between light and dark.

The contrasts in life showed me; without the painful and dark experiences I would never have fully understood the joy and light. I was now willing to confront the darkest corners of my pain. It is only when the darkness is exposed to the light the colours appear. Then I can see the whole picture and my unconscious mind slowly is able to let go of what it has tried to hide and forget for all these years. To protect me from being overwhelmed, my dreams give me symbols (pictures or parables) of the painful memories. Then I can interpret the dream as I am willing and ready to process it. The ego does not help me in this work. It resists all the changes and is in no way interested in releasing the memories, because it will then loose the grip on my life as I know it. Maybe it is why we so easily forget our dreams as soon as we wake up? To trick the ego attempting to prevent me from remembering or understanding myself, the 'dreamer', my sub-consciousness uses symbols and signs. *Funny,* I thought, and felt a bit smarter than my ego every time I was able to understand the underlying message of my dream.

When the cause of the painful memories is exposed, the pain (the symptom) can be healed. Wisdom is the gift resulting from a recognised and healed experience. Life was using every means possible to try to communicate with me. I was now encouraged to look even closer at my self-image.

A symbol is the shape created as the conscious and unconscious meet. The word for consciousness in German is 'Sinnbild'. It is a meeting between the mental, male facet of the soul and the female, creative facet. As I tried to 'read' the image of myself looking back I remember as a child the Africans called me 'Gole' that means big cheeks. I have always been smiling with my big round cheeks. I ponder the fact that my big cheeks reflect the inner strength and joy that I do possess and started to understand I had to *see myself* with eyes of love. I had to be willing to acknowledge my beauty and strength, but I faced great resistance from my ego. What if I ended up becoming too big and too beautiful? The ego never stopped.

Astrology and Archetypes.

We truly have been given the tools and help to recognise who we really are. I was awakened to the unconscious relationship with myself in earnest when I discovered astrology. It was yet another valuable gift I stumbled upon on my journey. Astrology is a mirror and tool we have received to find our way in our inner universe. The stars show the macro-cosmos reflected in my inner micro-cosmos at the moment I was born, like a fingerprint. In the astrological image I can find the outline of the potential and challenges I am faced with, as well as the gifts I have been given to take along to enhance my awareness.

The first meeting with astrology became a tough encounter. I got a knock-out I had not expected. The ego was protesting wildly. Still, I quickly discovered there was something there I had to face. I learned when we react strongly and emotionally to something, it is often because it reflects something in us that we do not want to reveal or see. The ego squirmed; it did not want to be exposed. Everything shown to me was painful recognitions. Astrology became an important guide and I learned to 'follow the stars'.

Astrology seen from the perspective of the soul shows us there are four main forces in our world and our soul has come to earth to experience itself through experiencing how these four forces beauty, joy, love and wisdom play out.

– Per H. Gullfoss

Psychiatrist Carl Gustav Jung also used the astrological map as a starting point with his clients.

This was not much publicised as it was of course not accepted amongst his colleagues in the West. Astrology really shows science and metaphysics are two sides of the same coin and complement each other. Jung was also very fascinated with dream work and encouraged everyone to learn the 'dream language'.

Whether you believe in astrology or not, I personally experienced everything I saw in my natal chart was amazingly recognisable and very revealing. As I opened the window to this inner universe, I was soon pulled deep into this fascinating source of knowledge. In astrology, your birthday or sun sign tells you about your life mission. The sun sign indicates what you are to do and develop. Has anyone guessed me to be a Capricorn at this point? Yes, sure I was born in the sign of Capricorn. The stubborn never giving up Capricorn! The ones who push stones uphill, without any other reason than 'life is supposed to be hard'.

It is the sign representing ambition, endurance and responsibility, but also mystical searching. The Capricorn is to learn how to put one brick upon another in building his life, and in doing this also trusting all the Universe has part in the process. I am to learn responsibility and patience and trust to open to support, joy and beauty in everything around me. Really, it is all about bringing light to matter. All astrological signs have a shadow side – a challenge. A Capricorn often thinks he must do everything on his own – and preferably reach the highest mountain peak. This often makes the journey difficult and painful. If you learn to see the help and tools that are available to you at birth, your life will become far easier and much more fun.

The help is truly everywhere.

Where the moon in the sky at the time of birth, symbolises the emotional gifts we are given from birth. In my birth chart the moon is in Sagittarius. This energy is outgoing, truth seeking and impatient. It has an eternal optimist energy, but the problem is he thinks everything needs to be done yesterday. Things can go so fast for a Sagittarius that one easily can stumble or lose track of the goal.

The energy constellations between the sun and the moon in my birth chart show an obvious inner conflict of interests. I can therefore easily become my own worst enemy. The opposing sides therefore must learn to work together. As my life have been mirroring to me, I must take one-step at a time, listen and balance all extremes in my personality. I had been showed this before in the dream when walking the painful path of contrast (Chapter 2: Dream nr 3: The path of contrasts), as well as the dream where Mum and Dad's contrasting differences were illustrated in their black and white dresses (Chapter 6: Dream nr 5: In a large old house). To learn how to create harmony within myself is something that seems I needed to be reminded of time and again.

Code and numbers.

I had always been very preoccupied with creating harmony around me but had neglected to pay attention to my own inner unrest. It now insisted to be seen and heard. All resistance and every flight mechanism I had learned were images of my limited, arrogant and fearful ego. A way out of the pain could be found, but then I first had to expose my inner adversary. This challenge led me further into the mystery of the symbolic world.

Our natal chart also has a numerological fingerprint of the universe. Numerology is part of the metaphysical heritage the humanity brings along. Astrology and numerology work together naturally but parted ways to become separate disciplines only 300 years ago. They were used together for thousands of years before astrology was rejected as a science and numerology became a secret tool only for the initiated. Although, the knowledge had existed through immemorial times, it was rediscovered and made available to us in the West by the great mathematician Pythagoras. Mathematics and numbers embody beauty and harmony which the great artists have included in their creative process through centuries. System is created from chaos with this tool. Beauty is harmony, and harmony is love.

Beauty will save the world.

– Fjodor M. Dostojevskij

Several esoteric writings that were part of the Bible also include the knowledge of numbers. The church and clergy knew these writings carried knowledge to inspire independent thinking and free choice, equality and therefore also inspired the right to create and choose how they wanted to live. This scared the people in power so much that they removed this information from the sacred writings. Thankfully, several of these originally hidden and forgotten writings have now reappeared. These scripts also tell us of wisdom presenting greater tolerance and acceptance of the human as being co-creator. We are now about to wake up to this power within which also means a great responsibility.

The number 26, which is my birthday, in numerology stands for the healer who has the tendency to help others at their own expense. One who has great power but must learn to use it in balance and cooperation with its surroundings as well as everything with the Higher self. Here I noticed something. If I fail myself, I fail everything. This is exactly what I had always done! I realised to sacrifice oneself was not a very pretty virtue. This only created abusers – people who exploited me. I had to realise I am worthy. This was a recognition that was very contrary to what the church had taught me. I had heard from the pews all through my childhood that I was but dust, and how small and insignificant I was. For years, I thought it was blasphemous to think I was anything more than dust, but something deep inside told me something different.

As a child I had a personal relationship with Jesus, but I thought I was not sure if the grown-ups really understood Jesus. I had to become an adult before I could embrace what was my 'Godly heritage', unconditional love! Still, it was a difficult process to acknowledge and accept the beautiful colours inside of me. Was I truly allowed to think I was a beautiful soul? Am I allowed to believe I am deserving of love and deserve the best? It seems to be a big challenge for all of us to recognise our inner light and beauty. I almost felt it was a sin to acknowledge and honour my own wishes and dreams. I came to the world with many gifts but to truly accept them was painfully difficult.

The colours of the rainbow.

As a young mother of 24 years old I applied for Art School in Oslo. Out of old habit I thought I really could not consider the best options, the one I really wanted. I therefore applied where everyone thought I would have the greatest chance of being admitted. I studied to become a ceramist while envying the ones painting. I knew how to draw but was not sure if I could paint. Better not aim too high. A teacher in high school once told me I was clever in drawing, but I did not have colour perception. I believed him and denied myself what I really wanted to become – a painter. I once again listened to the voice which confirmed my poor self-image.

After finishing ceramic studies, I opened a studio and business with a friend. I turned large tableware and pots and played with the décor as if the clay was a canvas. I painted female bodies leaping across the dish and it turned to be quite successful. One day as I was turning an exceptionally large dish which required much strength and skill, I disclosed my unconscious intention. Suddenly, I discovered the real reason for me to turn up this large dish was to be able to paint and play the decoration into being. Finally, I was ready to admit I wanted to become a painter. My desire to paint had finally managed to get through to my awareness. I wondered what else I was blind to or kept back. Strange how we play hide and seek with ourselves throughout much of our lives. How many detours did I need to take to find joy and happiness?

I returned to art school at 28 years old and studied a couple of years more. Doing painting, and I rediscovered the joy and passion of it. Nothing was wrong with my colour perception, my tutor and artist, painter Egil Weigelin said, as he watched me paint. In fact, it really was terrific, he encouraged me. Now, I learned how to play with the colours and learned their power and meaning. This eventually became my strength; to join the artist in me with my intuition strengthened the mystic ability. Later, when I started to conduct courses in intuitive painting, I learned this to be an amazing way to discover the unconscious. I could often read the individuals' story in the lines, shapes and colours. Intuitively, we all communicate everything that is within – like a fingerprint. I discovered I could read what my pupils expressed in their drawings. I understood I had the gift 'to see'.

Colours express the quality of the seven invisible energy centres in the body, the rainbow bridge connected to chakras. Like the arch of the rainbow the colours move up the spine throughout the body, like a big magnetic energy field. Each chakra is also symbolically tied to the four elements, water, earth, air and fire. The fifth element is spirit and is situated in the higher chakras on top of the head. Knowing about the energy centres, their colours and purpose is a great aid in dream work.

If I in my dream find myself in a house which often symbolises our lives, the level I find myself on in the house often show which stage in my life I am dreaming about. It shows what emotions dominate this level and what element is influencing me. It takes time and effort to learn 'the God language', the universal language of symbols. I studied everything I could lay my hands on to understand what my dreams were trying to tell me and to understand my inner map. I wanted to expose why I had not felt worthy of good things, realising I needed to break this pattern as soon as possible.

Crystals and knowledge.

One night, I received a dream (Chapter 8: Dream nr 10: A tomb in India) where I was standing outside an empty tomb in India. It was a cave carved out of a light ochre-coloured mud wall. It was half-full of dark water. I picked up beautiful crystals and gemstones that were scattered outside the cave and put them in a small red velvet bag. To the left, I could see an old Indian guru. He gave me a large green emerald. It was shaped like a pyramid. As I was holding it in my hand, it changed into a crystal-rod formed as a rectangle prism. On two sides, this emerald was covered with dried mud. I saw a story had been engraved as a relief on the mud. The old guru told me he would die within half an hour. "Two kings have owned this stone," he added cryptically.

I woke up feeling good but still at a loss. It seemed like an important dream and somehow, I felt an urgency about it. What in the world is it that I do not understand? What am I supposed to do with this stone and why the hurry? I obviously had gifts which I was not conscious of or using yet. Slowly, it dawned on me the gifts seem too big for me! I did not feel worthy. I moved into a quiet, deep meditation. I breathed in deeply and breathed out all critical thoughts. This is simply the ego trying to prevent the awakening, I knew. I had to reset my system into a neutral state before returning to the dream.

Then, instinctively 'old knowledge' popped up. The king represents great authority. This authority which I have been so very scared of, I now have to acknowledge. The large emerald symbolises pure old knowledge, success and healing. Green is the colour of the heart and tells me, everything must happen through the heart. My heart needs to heal and learn to trust. I must learn to receive as much as to give. In the dream, the emerald was first shaped like a pyramid, symbolising old, pure wisdom and joy. The emerald then changed to a form of a crystal-rod, which stands for manifestation and authority. I am supposed to manifest Joy, Beauty, Love and Healing.

India symbolises old wisdom. Capricorn is also the astrological sign for India. As mentioned, this sign represents authority, responsibility, endurance and a strong occult power. The crystals and gemstones I had picked up were knowledge and spiritual wisdom I had brought with me from Eastern philosophy. The water in the tomb was stagnant. This could symbolise old feelings that had not been released but carried through generations. This dream could also have a message for the general public. The old emotions gained through earlier experience are poisoned and must be cleaned, forgiven and released. I cannot allow previous mistakes and fears to stand in the way of my inner authority and true joy, my inner Sun.

My story, or our common history, was written in the clay covering the two sides of the stone. This can be washed away to make the gem, the knowledge, clean and pure again. We do not need to carry along our stories if the learning is integrated. I need the courage to become visible and let go of the 'pain story', take responsibility and share the joy inside. I need to integrate my authority and take the stage.

The dream continues to grow within. I have not yet learned to accept the greatness within and dare not identify with it. I deserve to receive the best – it is my Godly heritage. In fact, I have a responsibility to bring the dream to light. But oh, so hard to take that to the heart.

Gifts of my life.

My children are the most precious jewels in my life. They reflect gifts and challenges that I need to accept within myself. Every time I was pregnant, I felt a big light inside. I was happy and strong, and people said I was glowing. I knew it was true because that was exactly how I felt – every time. As I held my firstborn, it was evening and dark outside. I still felt the sun was shining, and I could hear birds singing outside my window. I was sure an angel was born. He was happy and content all day long. At school, he used humour to avoid fights, his teacher told me. As an adult, he is a rock to all who need his help and reflects goodness and a great sense of responsibility. I was reminded to strengthen and balance these qualities within myself.

Six years later, on a sunny Sunday morning I sat holding my beautiful daughter. The delivery had been quick and easy. She was in a hurry to enter the world. She showed me a playful, vulnerable and creative temperament with a powerful determination. I needed to mirror this as well. She holds great resources and defies the fear within by taking on challenges. I see these areas in myself that need to be strengthened and say, 'thank you'.

Another six years later, my youngest child was born. A big, strong and happy boy with a good sense of humour. He is not tongue-tied with his wit and talkative nature. He sees through untruth and dares to say so. He inspired me to play, to be truer to myself and to express myself clearly. I cannot contain my gratefulness for these gifts.

Then still later the grandchildren arrived on the scene. I thank the universe for these colourful and sparkly jewels. They colour my life in beautiful ways and the rainbow in my life shines stronger and purer.

Chapter 9
The Thread

The ego will have us chasing our tails.

– Dr Peeble

I had to sit quietly and take one day at a time. I was grateful for what have been revealed to me, all the gifts of my story. The stillness was truly a blessing. I had been excluded from the busy and stressful world around me to discover who I truly am and to find my life purpose. But it was not easy to surrender to the moment. Not at all. The Ego wanted me to "chase my tale" – my old story.

In my journal from this time, I found a dream (Chapter 9: Dream nr 11: A bundle of yarn) which was to show me an additional piece in the tapestry of my sub-consciousness. I dreamt I was going to join a seminar and was standing in the back of a packed auditorium. I looked around and could not find any free seats and got the feeling I just had to accept the fact that none would show up. In front of me, on the floor was a huge 'brown-reddish' bundle of yarn with many tangles. I understood that before getting a seat I had to undo all the tangles. I knew it would be a big and demanding job, but obviously had to simply accept it. I sat down a bit disheartened and faced the challenge. Then I woke up.

I love studying and teaching. Now, it was time to focus on learning about myself. Now, I had both the time and opportunity to engage in this work. The strong breakout of psoriasis had forced me to sit still. I could not stand on my feet without the skin cracking. Painting was impossible with all the lesions in my hands. Now, I was simply left with sitting still and going through the thread of history of my life. I learned to focus on what I had and not what I did not have. I had time…

The bundle in my dream represented the stories that follow us through our heritage. I understood the tangles were blockages in my psyche the thread represented the blood flowing through generations, a 'brownish-red' blood tie. Some patterns in my awareness were so deep-rooted they manifested in blockages in energy centres and vitally important functions of my body like the blood, breath, voice and heartbeat. The knots in the yarn represented unreconciled pain stories that had blocked the flow of life. The patterns had followed me through generations.

If I try to pull on the knots, they will only tighten harder. I had to sit down quietly with each tangle, breathe deeply and take the time necessary to untangle them. Meditation helped me with the patience, insight and love I needed to see what each tangle contained, and how I could lovingly release them. This was no mental exercise but rather an exercise in self-love. I had to lovingly recognising the fear and acknowledging patterns that had been formed through time. One of my many thought patterns was regarding worry concerning money, so naturally I received an exercise to teach me about this. One day, I was going to meet up with a friend. It was her birthday and she had invited me for a coffee. I discovered that all I had to my name was 50 Kroners. This was all I had to live on during the following week. I passed by a flower shop where they advertised a beautiful bouquet of flowers for 49 Kroners. There was nothing I could do to make it through the next week in keeping the money, so I bought the flowers and said a prayer, "Now, I need help to make it through the rest of the month." We had a lovely time-sharing a cup of coffee at her place and my friend was so happy to receive the flowers. As I returned home later that day, I discovered a cheque in the mail for several hundred kroners. It was a return for a bill I had unknowingly paid twice. I quietly sighed and said "thank you".

The lack of money was at that instance a knot that I did not tighten by worrying. Worry is a fear energy which constricts. But my life is reminding me of something important: I am not alone. Somebody is listening to me.

My intuition is like a glowing street sign. It knows and understands which pattern, thread or path I must recognise and which knots or resistance I am ready to release. It was a work in self-love, willpower and patience to persist in this process.

Indian shamans honour traumas and crises as portals to ones' Source. They look at every 'pain story' as gifts, revealing to us our 'unused power'. Crises, wounds or illness create a spiritual breakthrough and is a sign that the 'Great Spirit' has chosen you to perform a greater task. Therefore, they respect the ones who do not give up but continue as a light worker. There is no shame in being ill, on the contrary it is a possibility for growth and awakening. The elders tell stories with symbols and metaphors that can help the sick person on their journey and stand with them to help in the healing.

Since we do not live in such a communal society, I had to ask for help from a 'wise woman' here in Norway. Art therapist and healer Kaja Finne who had helped me previously became again my saving angel. She asked me to draw the girl inside as well as of the mature woman. I was asked to draw intuitively – with an open heart. I quickly drew a thin, tall girl in a dress, standing alone on a vast savanna. I looked at the picture and sensed that she was not afraid. She was secure, although alone. I wanted to rediscover her.

When I intuitively drew the 'mature woman', the one I wished to be, it turned out to become a wonderfully beautiful woman. She was pink, thriving, naked and with no hair. Around her chest, I saw thousands of glowing colour particles. I was astonished to see what I had created, and at the same time I realised that this was me – yet unknown, on a different level. I had never seen her either in my dreams, or visions before. She just appeared there and then.

The pictures I had created at this point set the awareness process in motion. Something had been planted. It was about something greater and more beautiful that no one had told me about before. Today I know the naked head means she has given up her personal and collective pain-story. All the colour particles floating around my chest and heart symbolised aspects of joy, creation and healing energies. She is naked, showing that she is honest and no longer has anything to hide. It was a dream version of myself – some time way into the future I told myself. Kaja Finne also asked me to draw three portraits of myself. I was to make some quick sketches not trying to make them look like anything special, she said. It became three quite different versions of what I at times think I am. I sketched intuitively and so quickly that my ego was not able to evaluate or judge it. You can trick your ego in this way! One of the portraits showed a critical, stern face which most likely tried to hide some fear. I did not like the sight of her but knew that she was there, and I had to love her into freedom. Then I saw a strong and happy face that wanted the best for everyone. I knew her. I had a hard time remembering the third face, most likely because this was the face that I did not know yet – and I was about to learn to know her.

The drawings were signs from my higher self. I leave fingerprints in everything I create and think. As an artist I have often later discovered important traces in my artwork of things I was not yet ready to acknowledge at the time I painted it. Everything within and around us tries to awaken us to be healed and happy. In the book, 'The Medicine of the Consciousness' written by Gill Edwards, she convincingly describes and documents how the body reacts to thoughts and feelings. She was a psychologist and author of several books where she challenged the current conventional medicine. Her insight and work have received recognition from several of today's premier doctors and scientists. Gill Edwards worked with the question, "Is illness always an expression of dissatisfaction?" Her conclusion was yes.

I tried to listen more closely to the signals of my body. All the way through to mature age I had struggled with my breath. I would breathe shallowly throughout the day, and at night my throat would contract, cramping to the point that I could not breathe. The fear created tension in my body, which again blocked the free flow of energy and therefore activated the emergency alarm. What was I so afraid of? Breath is life. Was I afraid of Life itself?

I am dependent on breath to survive. It needs to flow freely as an ever-flowing river, as a thread without knots. I learned the breath is automatically guided from the brainstem and intricately connected with the brain's survival mechanism. If it stops, I die. When I experience danger, I will respond with activating the adrenalin which activates the fight or flight mechanism. An instinct which instructs the body to fight or escape to survive. The body is supplied with energy through increased pulse and adrenaline to survive and I engage in battle mode. If I regard this power as overwhelming, I will respond by freezing and automatically hold my breath. I realised I very often 'hold my breath'. It is the opposite action that will help me.

Here some wires were crossed for sure.

Breath is the Bridge which connects life to consciousness, which unites your body to your thoughts. Whenever your mind becomes scattered, use your breath as the means to take hold of your mind again.

– Thich Nhat Hanh

The chain is never stronger than its weakest link, they say. I cannot survive without air, and therefore the breath becomes my weakest link. The paradox is it is also my greatest power of manifestation. The breath connects me with life and is a bridge between the spirit (Source) and matter (the body). I had to relax and open to the life-force.

When I relaxed my breath was flowing. So, what was stressing me? What was holding my breath captured? Often memories of old fears hidden within can be triggered and we react as if the circumstances are real – in the moment. I learned this is but an unprocessed memory being awakened. We think we are in the same situation as way back at the same moment when the memory was made. I had to reprogram this old memory to allow the body to let go of the reaction. If I take the time and breath through this process, just like when going through labour, the fear is released. Meditation became especially important in aiding my breath to flow unrestricted.

To my surprise, I discovered the breathing problems are quite common! I found this to be strange since breathing is so fundamental to existence.

When I at last was able to open and let the breath flow, the tears would come. It was like a powerful opener to my emotions. If I want to live, I must breathe. If I want to love, I must open my heart. If I want to be heard I must pick up the courage to use my voice and express my desire in words. If I want to be free, I must let go of fear. What it all comes down to is a choice between fear or love.

What you resist will persist. I read this somewhere. I think we have enough organisations and institutions whose aim is to fight *against* something, like the war against AIDs, the war against terror and so on. A journalist once asked Mother Theresa if she would support the fighting against AIDs. With a warm smile, she answered, "If I am asked to be for something, I'll support it." I think we often get stuck in negative thought patterns of always being 'ready for battle' and on guard. This leads to believing in resistance to everything. Then we get overwhelmed with stress. We are continually on guard and eventually it will create chronic tension in our muscles, which eventually becomes inflammation when the body is exhausted.

The picture was starting to take shape. Slowly, I could see I really needed to let go of all my old thinking pattern. Awareness or consciousness is light, they say. I was helped by the light within as I breathed through the layers of dark shadows without resisting them. As in the fairy-tale, the troll bursts when the rays of sunshine hit it. The troll, pattern, habit or knot dissolves when the light of awareness reaches it.

My voice and breath are linked together and are both strong channels of manifesting. At this time of my process I was a member of a choir in Oslo. Here, I learned to know a gifted musical teacher, Lulle Sandemose, a beautiful and wise soul. She became my saving angel as she took me in and tutored me. I desperately needed to set my voice free and for three years, I did breathe exercises with Lulle. I really did not sing much but still my voice loosened and its power and depth was discovered. What surprised me the most was the terrible fear I experienced, faced with allowing my voice to be set free. Lulle did not give up on me that easy, and thanks to her patience and motherly strength I was able to break through the resistance within me. My voice became strong, pure and vibrant. It both shocked me as well as made me incredibly happy. Suddenly, I was asked if I would like to try as a soloist in a Christmas oratorio. The blockages from childhood had loosened. I obviously was not alone on this journey of life. The universe sent me all the help that I needed if I just was willing to step on to the stage.

I was continually searching for new insights and gifts hidden inside of me. Maybe it was traumas needing a 'hiding place' till the time was right to deal with them? I was looking at every possibility. The well-known shaman, therapist and author Sandra Ingerman, writes about the loss of parts of the soul in her book *Soul Retrieval*. After studying this phenomenon, I tried this retriever technique through a wake dream-work. I let go of all control to allow for a deep and relaxing meditative state and then called on my 'helper', who in this case showed up as a lioness. I asked the lioness to take me along to the place where my pain was hiding so I could release it. I allowed her to lead me up and way into a mountainous area. Dusk was settling, and the journey went on and on. I started to wonder if it was necessary for the journey to take so long. Finally, it seemed we had arrived. We were standing way up on top of a mountain right in front of an opening to a cave. I waited patiently, as I instinctively knew I had to. Suddenly, a huge green dragon came out of the cave. It towered above me and seemed very threatening and irritated by the disturbance. I was forced to avail myself of a strength I did not think I possessed. With the authority worthy of a lioness I demanded for the dragon to return what it had taken from me. My intention was so strong and clear that the dragon had no choice. My word was its command! The dragon opened his mouth, huge and red and with a roar spit out a little child that came tumbling down on the ground in front of me. Surprised, I quickly picked up the child and backed off into safety. The lioness, child and I returned home.

As I opened my eyes, I felt a deep and all-encompassing relief, amazement and thankfulness. The lion is a symbol of solar plexus, the third chakra situated in the diaphragm, and is the seat for strength and self-esteem. This aspect of me, led me to the hiding place of 'the monster', the deepest pattern that I was so fearful of. The dragon, my monster had hidden what was dearest from me. The inner child had to be released through the throat, the fifth chakra, which is the centre for manifestation, where we express our willpower. The child, the symbol for the heart, where dreams reside, had been trapped by fear all these years.

I had never dared to express my opinions and had therefore not fought for or defended my inner child. Finally, I dared to take back my power. My throat was opened, and the child could express itself freely.

Through childhood and adolescence my strategy for survival had been to stay quietly in the background. If I lay low, I would not create any waves. *Then everyone would be happy,* I thought. "If you don't dare to make waves, you'll drown," the psychologist told me. I understood this picture. Now, I had to dare to create waves.

I had to muster up all the willpower I could in the long and difficult process of getting the support and help I needed from the establishment, where there were personal agendas and accountings to balance. Despite all the inner work that I had done, the physical ailments were prolonged, and I had to face the fact that my condition made it impossible for me to work. Together with my doctor, phycologist and a wise lawyer I received great help. I knew we would finally have a breakthrough because I had no other option. I could not let myself down any longer. A deep-rooted pattern finally unravelled when I picked up the courage to start fighting for myself. Resolve follows faith! I had to fan the flame of my dreams and look to the future. If you do not know where you want to go, there is no use in wishing your way forward. I knew where I wanted to go and did not let go of the horizon, where my dream castle was gleaming in the sun. Hope is the light shone on the road forward, I had learned.

My deceased grandmother came through for me with a message through a channelling session with the medium Christine Argent, who was visiting Oslo. The venue was crowded with people coming to experience her channelling. Unexpectedly, she turned to me. My grandmother came through to ask why I had not started doing what I wanted to do yet. She specifically mentioned the use of colours. The medium knew nothing about me and therefore could not have known that I was a painter. Grandma also asked me to go on a vacation. That got me quite annoyed, because I did not have any money, although I had thought about it a lot. *Didn't they get it on the other side,* I thought wryly. Then the medium turned to my friend sitting next to me. Her mother who died when she was only a young girl, came through. Her mother first had an important and personal message for her, and then she asked if she could address me. Surprised, I received a heartfelt thank you from this deceased stranger for the support that I had been to her daughter. This was very emotional for both of us as we listened and moved said thank you.

A few months later, surprisingly enough, I had the money and got a vacation. I was reminded we exist on various levels of existence, and I really am not alone. There is no death, only a new life, she had said! I started to realise fear was wasted energy. The tangles of life can more easily be undone when I let go of fear. The blood could flow more freely when my heart opens itself to life. I boldly pressed my ear a little closer to the pulse of life.

One evening a friend was visiting. We were going to practice healing on each other. When we were done, I laid there relaxing while enjoying the feeling of the blood rushing freely through my body. For a moment, the ancestral blood run through me, unrestricted and cleansed. Suddenly beautiful healing music came from my cd player. We had been working in silence for three hours and neither of us had touched the player. I looked at my friend and laughed. This had happened before but never with a witness present.

Chapter 10
Letting Go

Life was never meant to be a struggle, just a gentle progression from one point to another, much like walking through a valley on a sunny day.

– Stuart Wilde

A friend one day visited bringing a dream (Chapter 10: Dream nr 12: Covered with pollen) for interpretation. She dreamt she had been out for a walk and had to wash her feet when returning home. They were covered in pollen. She thought this was a strange and funny dream.

Pollen is a fitting symbol for something that impacts us if we are receptive. If we are receptive to something in our environment we will be "pollinated" by it, and then carry this forward. We only become immunised against the effect when we get rid of the receptor which is the expectations created by the pain body. That is the part of us that expects something unwanted or wanted will happen again, and because of this expectation it is reactivated.

Later in the day, my friend phoned me. She was concerned she had 'infected' me with her bad mood while visiting. I laughed stating that it had not affected me at all. There was no 'receptor' in me that day so we both had a good laugh. I was reminded it is possible to avoid being affected if you are consciously present in yourself at that moment. It is not necessarily easy, but it is possible. I was learning something new every day.

The illness had led me into an unending and mystical universe. There were lots to learn here, and many questions were answered if I allowed myself to be present and give myself the time to interpret and read all the signs that appeared.

I was willing to confront more of my addictions and illusions as time was going by. At this point, I had a dream (Chapter 10: Dream nr 13: Give birth to a baby) where I was together with a couple of friends. They wanted me to give birth to a baby. We all sat dressed in a large white bed. After I had reluctantly let myself be convinced, I suddenly had a new-born, naked little baby in my arms. I held the baby feeling confused and a bit disheartened when the baby suddenly changed to a round and smooth shape that slipped out of my hands and onto the floor. This felt like a hopeless task I had been given – or had taken on. As I woke up, I felt this was a warning.

In this dream, I had been reminded of an old pattern where I often take responsibility for something that really is not mine to deal with. In the safe meditative space, I was able to explore this old pain-body. My biggest challenge is to let go of people who give the impression of 'needing' me. Often it might be right to help somebody, but for some reason this time I felt unsettled about it. I think I felt manipulated. Taking responsibility for how others feel is the most difficult pattern for me to break. My ego had lived and thrived on being needed by others, from my childhood, even if it implied disallowing my own needs.

The dream gave me a clear answer to a dilemma I had put myself into. The child represented a project which was not mine. My friends had asked me to participate in their work, but it did not feel right for me at that time. I thankfully let go of the situation and felt light and free. Slowly I learned to relax and release…

I was now 55 years old and had finally started to feel things were moving in the right direction – even though slowly. My body was still hanging on to all the symptoms, but now I had a much brighter outlook on life. Thankfully, I had a couple of faithful friends to lean on during this time. They were not afraid to mirror things to me or see themselves in my reflection. Our exchanges were honest and very needed and helpful. Still, I also wanted seclusion and quiet to help me see things clearer. One day I heard, "You have to detach from the collective consciousness." This sounded completely unreasonable to me. But it started to be a bit clearer what this entailed. I had to distance myself from my own and other 'stories' and dramas.

Distance aids both in getting a greater overview as well as further insight. I learned to look at every experience as a Story. All experiences are gifts and if I 'rewrite' these into mythical stories and symbols, they will show the deeper meaning and wisdom that my experience is gifting me with. When I turn the experience into an impersonal image, story or parable, the ego is not as easily engaged in the process, and it will be easier to let go.

Dreams continued to guide me. I asked, and the dreams often rewarded me with answers. The more I listened the clearer they became. One day, I struck up a conversation with a young man who was considering returning to visit Cameroon in Africa, the country I grew up in. A few years earlier, he had been teaching at the primary school in Ngaoundere, where I had once been a student. He was wondering if I would be interested in coming along. My first reaction was that maybe I should, but then I started sensing a strong discomfort and I asked for a little time to consider it. I discovered I was quite proud of myself for asking of this. Because of my desire to please, doing so had not been easy for me in the past.

That following night I dreamt (Chapter 10: Dream nr 14: Outside of a high wall) I was standing on the small bridge leading up to the mission station in Ngaoundere. I was surprised to see it was now surrounded by a high mud wall. I know it had not been there before. Right in front of me I saw a large and heavy wooden door that was closed. I did not think I could open it. Suddenly, I found myself floating up above the wall and looking down on the other side. To my surprise, I discovered more walls on the inside creating a large labyrinth. I did not feel I would like to go there.

I did not even need to meditate when I woke up to understand this dream. It was a large and clear 'stop' sign and I did not go to Cameroon. Maybe I will some time, but this was obviously not the right time. I was able to decline the offer and felt a bit freer from the past. Now was the time to continue the inward journey. The silence magically opens windows inward to reveal forgotten memories. As I was focused, my inner light had been turned on and I was slowly finding my way in my inner landscape.

I was now reminded of the mystery of how our subconscious can create and connect with us through the tool of intuitive painting. For years, I had been teaching in this wonderful art and found it was an excellent key to enter the locked rooms inside of us. It connects us to the levels that we are not consciously able to reach. It is another way of dreaming.

One fun example to illustrate how this happened is when I was asked to give a lecture and a creative presentation at an inspirational seminar for the employees at the executive board of the government department for Health and Social Affairs.

I asked the participants to paint a tree without premeditation. Then I asked if they would allow me to analyse each tree. They all were entertained and amused by the fact that I could read so much about every one of them simply from the tree they had painted. One person had instinctively managed to include her own unique hairdo much to her own amusement as well as the rest of the assembly. With our unique fingerprint, we mirror and express who we are in everything we think and do, whether we are aware of it or not. It is really a waste of energy to think we can hide who we are. The quest we must do is to figure out ourselves and our purpose for life. That we cannot do by hiding…

I consistently had used meditation as a door opener in my sessions. The attendants were helped to let go of all their expectations and performance anxiety before exploring and expressing themselves with colours. Expectations can be an extraordinarily strong critical energy because it carries the idea of a specific outcome and the idea that something is more important or right than something else. Expectations can create fear which again blocks the process of creation. Meditation helps loosen all resistance and creates peace and safety to support a playful joy of creating. One must 'Relax' to 'Release' and then be able to 'Receive'.

One day, while still at my centre, a woman arrived and asked for help. She had discovered art as a transformative energy to help her with a drug addiction she had suffered from much of her young life. The problem was she now had a drought in her creative work and did not know what to do to get going again. She proudly showed me a few slides of her paintings. Technically they were incredibly good, but when I 'tuned' into her energy I discovered a 'black hole' in her childhood. When I confronted her with this insight, she confirmed I was right. I asked her if she would be willing to join in on a couple of sessions of our intuitive painting workshop to possibly help her open the closed room inside of her. She could try it out without cost and without committing to the whole workshop, I offered her. The only thing that was required of her was to take this chance and let go of her need to control. If she wanted to join the workshop, she had to dare to release her inner child for a while, I told her. But she did not dare.

She was able to master the techniques that she had control over, and through this she thought she had found her identity. She did not understand her inner child was trapped in the techniques, 'the achiever,' and this created blockage which again dried up her flow of creative energy. The expectations she had of herself to create the 'perfect' picture had to be released. She had to experience she was good enough without linking it to any type of achievements. As she left, her eyes showed hurt and fear. She was too scared to follow the sign pointing to freedom and chose to turn back to her known path, her comfort zone. I never met her again. Indeed, to receive we must release.

I could see the reflection of myself in this story and discover the source of my own fear of failure. 'Kill your darlings' is an expression I used much when teaching. Now, I had to be willing to let go of the 'dearest and nearest' to be able to move on. What we are good at can very soon become our Achilles heel. Was I taking myself too seriously? Was I too attached to the outcome? Was I keeping my sun and power locked up for fear of not being perfect?

When I was able to paint freely and without fear, all the paintings became lighter, brighter and cheerier. Seriousness, which often is caused by fear-based and self-important thoughts, loosened its grip and I was liberated to create. Everything my memories showed me now, were all mirroring what I was ready to process and let go of. I was guided in every step.

My experience as a teacher in the Norwegian school system reflected how priorities in society at large can hurt the child within. The curriculum put strict and limiting restrictions as a framework for what I was supposed to teach in arts and crafts. I realised what I could have given the children, and I knew the approach to inspire their creative growth, But I was stopped in every attempt that could in any way deviate from the strict agenda put in place. When the curriculum stresses a certain task is to be done in a particular way and within a certain timeframe and with limited resources, creativity dies. The fear of losing control and not being able to produce yearly estimates, cause the elected to simply overlook the basic factors of the individual child's needs and therefore the mental and fear-based culture wins, and the creative child loses. When we continuously compromise, our identity is gradually wounded. This goes for the whole society as well as for me. I had to take care of my own inner child now.

If we could see the miracle of a single flower clearly, our whole life would change.

– Buddha

Children are like growing flowers. They need nurturing, care, respect and to meet their individual needs and conditions for thriving. The universe was mirroring back to me what I needed to see. To learn about myself, I just had to look around me.

Some years ago, I was heading up a pilot program. It was initiated by the municipality and we were to try out if there would be a base and interest for a broader and permanent creative proposal for the children in this district in Oslo. Students from 6th grade, picked from six different classes at the same school were to participate for six weeks. When all had settled down, I put on soft background music. Then I reminded them of the fact that there were no expectations linked to the outcome and that everything they created would be fine and good enough. They were also cautioned not to compare. Then I asked them to close their eyes, listen to the music and imagine they were in a warm and bright bubble, protecting them and giving them a nice, happy and safe feeling. After a short while sitting in this feeling, I asked them to open their eyes and start painting.

When the course ended, after six weeks, the results were so exciting that we decided to make a display at the school. We invited the local newspaper and all the teachers also came. The children received lots of encouraging attention and the teachers looked at the results with astonishment. A couple of them approached me and explained they had noticed in this short time there had been a strong increase in several of the students' performance level – and it was even noticeable in all subjects. They wondered if I could do a course with the teachers also. I was willing to do that, but they admitted there was no funding for such an initiative. Of Course!

When a child feels free, safe and is accepted, it will flourish and live out its potential. The creative child experiments and unceremoniously moves boundaries.

Albert Einstein thought imagination was far more important than knowledge. Imagination is owned by the free, searching and playful child. The inner child, our heart, knows and understands both the way and the signs. If I trust the child within, I must let go of the control. Then it will show the way and give me the key to my heart, my inner Sun and Power. The children are the dreamers who create the future.

Chapter 11
The Dreamer

If you want to remain always happy, always perfect and always fulfilled, then always keep inside your heart a pocketful of sweet dreams.

– Sri Chinmoy

The alchemist creates by believing he already is what he desires to create. He becomes one with his goal or dream. To manifest a dream requires that I must fully cooperate with the elements and energies of it. It demands I believe and feel I already am what I wish to be. The only thing that really exists is here and now. Magic can just happen in the moment.

The dream must be my own, not anything that is expected or coming from outside. It must be from my authentic self. One day, I came across something written by Vernon Howard. It is a conversation between God and a seeking soul, and it starts with a question to God. "I have been told that I need to believe in myself. Is that possible?"

God answered, "Who is this self you are talking about?"

The human answered, "I don't know."

Then God answered, "Then you have to be careful not to repeat popular sayings that you don't understand. If you, by myself, mean all the illusions you have accumulated about yourself, it would be dangerous to think this way. But if you mean your inner true self and original nature, it's a marvelous act to believe in the self."

We laugh and shake our heads at the dreamers amongst us. Anyway, I still decided to live out who I am – a naive dreamer. I lift my eyes, almost stubbornly towards the horizon – towards my dream. I had to find something else to focus on besides my hurting body. The pain and sores were not yet letting go. My feet still were very painful, so maybe I had to simply let go of my physical standing point? Maybe a trip away from all the 'Norwegian soberness' would do me good? At this moment, I was willing to try anything. I was not getting better by sitting in my 'safe' living room here in Norway any way. I did not take the cold and the dark winters well either. The voice in my heart faithfully stated its case, but I still had to accept waiting.

Slowly but surely, the little voice got through to me. Finally, I gathered the courage and strength and jumped on an airplane to the States. I took the Amtrak across the American continent, starting in New York. I got off in Chicago, where I stayed for three days before travelling on to Minneapolis. There I stayed with a friend a couple of days before I jumped back on the Amtrak. I spent two days and nights on the train, travelling through the enchanting Midwest toward Portland, which was my next destination. While on the train, I encountered beautiful and helpful people. They gave me the address to a perfect little and cheap hotel in Portland. I enjoyed a couple of weeks in a friendly, open, 'green' and 'alternative' environment. This gift of a journey continually gave me new insights and inspiration.

Again, I boarded the train and travelled south along the West Coast to San Diego, California. The sunshine and heat here nourished and warmed both body and soul, and slowly a new spark of life was ignited in me. That certain 'something' here had a positive effect on me both physically and emotionally. People were more open and warmer than I had experienced in Norway. Both my body and soul drank in every ray of sunshine and every smile as life-giving nectar.

Then came the time to return to Norway. The night before I boarded the plane, I had a dream (Chapter 11: Dream nr 15: Airplane crashes) where I was standing in an open field back in Norway. I saw a huge white airplane coming towards me from the right. I was frightened by how low it was flying and it then disappeared to the left behind a tall, dark pine forest. I heard a big crash and saw dark smoke rising. The smoke grew and soon covered the whole sky as a dark blanket. Then everything became dead quiet and dark. Fear was rushing through my body as I woke up.

I had to meditate to find the peace and comfort I needed to discover what this dream was all about. I took a deep breath and allowed all tension to leave my body as I exhaled and repeated this until I could feel everything was quiet inside. I turned my attention to the dream again and started working through all the different features shown. I felt most likely it was not a warning about an actual accident, but about the depression I had been struggling with in Norway. It could also be about a collective depression in the world economy as well, since I had the dream in late 2007. The fact that our dreams also can mirror something collective is not so unusual.

Airplanes symbolise thoughts and ideas, or high ambitions and visions. It was white which indicates a pure and happy vision. It came from the right side which indicates that the dream is about my future. The black smoke represents depression, thoughts that darken my mind when my dream about my future crashes. The hill with the tall pine trees represents Norway, for me. The dream was a strong warning not to allow my visions and dreams to crash when I returned to Norway. If so, the depression that I now had, and was slowly being released from, would take me again. The collective thought-energy in Norway was once again going to become a test. I was forewarned…

Do not allow your mind's cloud hover over your heart's aspiration-tree.
— Sri Chinmoy

Back in Oslo, I, one day, was sitting in a café. Two women from Nigeria were sitting to my right. It seemed an eternity since I lived in Africa. I felt starved. I could not let myself absorb the energy they were surrounded by. The women were full of life, warmth, passion and engagement. They played with gestures and words and did not shy away. They laughed, and their laughter rolled glibly around the room. A small grief settled on me. I really missed this. I missed this life force. It remined me of something still locked deep inside of me.

"Are you always so happy?" an elderly Norwegian lady asked me one day. I had finally become a grandmother and sat at the next table with my grandchild. Her question had a sharp undercurrent. I had been playing with and enjoying my grandchild while the lady watched us for more than an hour. She was out for a couple of hours to have a break from caring for her sick husband, she explained. It is hard to come to terms with others' joy if it does not live in oneself.

In the book 'The New Earth', Eckhart Tolle tells a story he has heard about people in the Nordic countries. "If you smile to a stranger on the street, you can get arrested for being drunk." This made me laugh. It is not really that bad, but it was interesting to note how others had experienced some of the same things I had noticed. Why aren't we happier and more grateful? I wondered if the reason could be that we are not allowing our self to Dream?

I was at my psychiatrist and was thinking out loud and relating my naïve dreams and ideals about the life I wanted to live. "Yes, just like Jesus," the psychiatrist remarked, sarcastically. Well, he truly was my role model, I thought amused and suddenly I burst into fits of laughter. I laughed at his tart commentary and could not stop laughing. Tears streamed down my cheeks as I laughed at the fact that what I so sincerely believed in was so utopic to him. It was as if we were on different planets. It is not easy to be an optimist in Norway. Are we really that cynical in this country? Are we that afraid of the dreamer inside – of our ideals? Are we so afraid of the light within? It seemed both pathetic and comical.

The gallows' humour in me awakened, and for a short moment I was a naked African who had nothing to hide. I had a good laugh while the psychiatrist thought I ought to cry. Oddly enough, the psychiatrist more than gladly digs through all the darkness with me but denies the light. You are not supposed to talk about it. Don't they believe in it? I was triggered…

As I returned to the next consultation the following week, he showed me proudly that he had insulated the wall to the next room. I understood my unconstrained laughter had embarrassed him. How Norwegian I thought sadly and did not see him again.

Why do we have to listen to our hearts? The boy asked. Because, wherever your heart is that is where you will find your treasure.
                                                            – Paulo Coelho

It was my life purpose to manifest the light within, I realised. I found we are more afraid of the light within than of the darkness. Thankfully, I still find many golden nuggets that daily inspire and light my way. I comforted myself with what feels right for me is also right for the whole.

I spent a lot of energy having to deal with my surroundings. They almost drowned me with their well-meaning advice and concerns. I really worked hard to stay afloat while despair and depression lurked around the corner. My strong desire to live a free and true life, and follow the impulses of the magician within, was continually warring with the deep fear of hurting or disappointing others. The body clearly showed I chose to hurt myself instead. I still struggled with an undefined feeling that I was responsible for other people's lives and wellbeing, and therefore ended up in a continual inner struggle regarding who I was to be there for. Did I really have the right to consider myself?

My intention to become a healthy and strong being had to be clarified. Was it because I wanted others to accept me or was it to help liberate the true me? Who was my taskmaster? Was it my ego or my higher self?

The well-known shaman, anthropologist and author Alberto Villoldo writes in *Courageous Dreaming* about 'Earthkeepers', shamans from the Andes and the Amazons who work to strengthen the intentions towards a peaceful new earth by dreaming it into being. They work vigilantly and consciously towards dreaming the new dream or the new world into existence *by giving it power through focus.* Their united effort will influence and manifest a new era and a better reality. These shamans do not allow for the egos to control the process. They ascend to a higher collective level of the soul group and make the intention a common cause, both for Mother Earth and every living thing.

I am not at that level yet and must concern myself with what I know and be loyal and faithful to my own dreams. I must live and breathe them as if they are real. I must dare to face the headwind and put the ego on a starvation regime.

Do not feed your ego and your problems, with your attention. Slowly, surely, the ego will lose weight, until one fine day it will be nothing but a thin ghost of its former self. You will be able to see right through it, to the divine presence that shines in each of us.

– Eknath Easwaran

Stress is most likely the common denominator for every symptom in my body. I had to learn to let go of everything that would cause it. Stress is a result of fear created by my ego. I saw the challenge was to not give it any more energy, focus or authority. I had to let go of my old stories that my ego was feeding on. *My ego was creating the stress to keep me where I was*. It did not want me to be a Dreamer, to dream new reality into my life.

I learned physical reactions are stored in our cells from the different experiences and memories we have. My only option to help change my body's responses was to create new peaceful thoughts and good memories. I had to dream into existence a new and better reality before I could be of help and give joy to the world. In the book *The Four Insights* Alberto Villoldo writes in Courageous Dreaming about the Indian shamans called Laika. They don't live according regular rules or norms; "if they wish to change anything in their world, they don't create new laws or promote new theories. Instead they choose to change their *perception* of the problem. Through changing their perception, they transform the problem to a possibility." I had to heal the perception of my life. Through meditation I received access to previous experiences and feelings outside of time and space. In this space I can recreate and heal both past and future when changing my perception of everything that has happened. The body believes everything I think and feel and cannot differentiate between imagined and actual actions or experiences. That is why it also does not differentiate between memories and today's reactions.

With new understanding I can create new attitudes that create a new reality.

The nightly dreams I had as a child living at the boarding school were often fearful. I would dream the floor was covered with crawling snakes, and I had nowhere to safely put my feet. Symbolically the snake belongs at the root chakra, which is the foundation for material and emotional safety. I felt insecure and unhappy because I lacked the safe foundation and framework that a home, with parents, gives. I did not trust this level. This insecurity was expressed physically by the fact that I continually sprained my ankle.

I now wanted to try to change my perception of these memories and feelings. Through a deep meditation I returned to these moments. I envisioned all was well and I was safely home with Mum and Dad. I stayed with the vision until I could feel my body had listened. Surprisingly, it worked. It gave me the feeling of being in safe hands. I was creating a new reality, a new perception of my childhood experiences into being. My body listened to these new thoughts, and it was easier to accept I was not trapped in my story. Strangely enough I hardly ever twist my ankle anymore.

Every time one of my dreams is giving me an animal, I always seek up the knowledge about the symbolic side of it. I found the snake is the symbol of transformation, from death to new life. The snake can both heal and kill and symbolises the ability to let go and shed the old skin (the identity). It tells us to let go of the past to give birth to a new life. In the traditions of the East, the snake is rolled up at the base of the spine, the first chakra, with a large and prevailing power. South symbolises where you stand, the physical reality we live in – the ground floor and our past. When this power is awakened it raises and ascends the spine as a pillar of fire or a rainbow. If you consider ancient wisdom and knowledge about this symbol, it is about sexuality, creativity, potent life force and transformation. This is powerful medicine, I thought. I am not my story and can let it go – as if it is an old cape.

I am not my experiences, but I own the experience and pain.

When I understood I could leave this old skin behind and stand up without fearing anything, my perception of my experiences was slowly changing. I am free to leave the story behind and move on. As this, positive thought has been given space in the subconscious, the process of healing has already started, but my ego yet fights the change.

Ego bravely defends its existence and its old and hard-earned stage in my life. If I let go of my 'skin', which symbolises my identity, I cannot count on gaining the acceptance of my surroundings. I might possibly not be recognised, and therefore must let go of my need for acceptance and recognition. This is of course challenging to the ego. I am also reminded that I am supposed to get out of the collective energy field. I must dare to stand-alone.

To be able to win this battle I must use tools that the ego does not control. *Meditation* puts the ego out of play for short spurts of time. Everything takes time and to me this is challenging. I feel I really should have arrived yesterday and to help me become more patient I had to work with my breath. I continually returned to this quiet room inside where all is well and where everything can be healed, dissolved and recreated.

The traditional work model psychologists often use is to allow the client to retell or re-experience everything that has caused pain. The Western therapy model does not have a tradition of how to deal with the process of letting go of old life patterns or memories of pain, the dying process. The focus is aimed backwards, so we walk with our backs towards the future. The gaze is turned away from the horizon and future and the hope glimmering ahead is ignored. What I have experienced is every story I retell awakens the emotions and recreates the energy of the experience. They reinforce the energy of the wounds. Every time I talk about and think about them, I give them nourishment and reactivate them. I have done this a lot.

Meditation helps me to break this pattern. Every time I meditate and allow the breath and light to envelope my thoughts, without expecting anything or trying to control it, I immediately feel better. Something happens automatically, as if the light within knows exactly what needs to be cleansed and removed. But the light can only work on the images or memories I am willing to let go of. The magic of the meditation is it does not make it painful to see and release the bad, as I stay safe in this quiet, bright space. After a while, the old thoughts received less attention and therefore less nourishment. My patterns of dependence were challenged to let go and slowly my thought patterns started to change. As a response to these changes my surroundings also started to let go of the restrains in my life.

Magic started to appear even more in my daily experiences. Life could be easy if I allowed it to be. If I only bless something the whole situation can neutralise and blockages dissolve.

Sometimes the pain I am faced with is even not mine, but it can give an opportunity for learning. I do not have to take on the drama of others.

The healer Kaja Finne taught me how I could bless a problematic situation or person by placing them in a pink bubble of light while putting myself in neutral energy. Then I was supposed to tell them, in my mind, not to harm me anymore and then blow away the bubble three times – up into the light. I was to do this for 3 days in a row, because repetition strengthens the intention. I had my first experience with this healing module at a seminar I attended. We were divided into smaller groups and I was placed in a group with three others. One of the attendants, a beautiful and strong woman, asked loudly not to be placed in the same group with me. "I don't trust her," she said and pointed towards me. She had not even talked with me. It was so absurd that I really could not take it personally. But I eventually started to feel that it was taxing to sense her negative feelings towards me. I did not want this to ruin an otherwise interesting seminar, so I decided to try what I had learned from Kaja Finne. The next morning while riding the bus to the next event I decided to try this healing technique. Three mornings in a row, I repeated the exercise and then forgot all about it. Strangely, I did not even notice that this woman was there. She sat three seats away from me throughout the whole seminar. At the end of eight weeks, when the event was ending, we all went around giving each other goodbye hugs and suddenly she stood there right in front of me. I was genuinely surprised. "Gro, can I give you a hug?" she asked as she cautiously walked towards me. I smiled and a little confused said "Yes".

She hugged me and whispered in my ear, "Thanks for showing me my strength!" I was shocked. It sure worked!

A therapist had suggested to her that maybe she was afraid of her own power, the power I had reflected. The thought she had created about me was only a projection of the fear she had towards her own strength. I had 'dreamt' this change into being by fully believing it to be possible. Life truly is filled of mysteries and 'reality' has many layers.

Chapter 12
A New Destination

Hope is at once both simple and profound. It is hope that binds heaven and earth.
Hope is the bridge between heaven and earth.

– Sri Chinmoy

In the classic illustration accompanying the Norwegian folks-tale about Ashlad, the gleaming fairy-tale castle is shining like gold in the horizon. The dream of gaining the princess and half the kingdom lives in us all. Ashlad, a poor courageous boy believed in his dream – and set out on his journey to find it. He was met with mockery and laughter, but he was the one who eventually realised his dream.

Thought creates, I am reminded of it again and again. I must create a vision of something better than my old story. Again, I was reminded that on a mystic level, I can somehow *rewrite my story*. My mind was lifted and started to focus on a brighter future.

The trip I had taken to the States had planted a seed of hope within me. The optimism and all the smiles warmed me deep inside. The weather also had a strong healing effect on me. I started allowing myself to dream of a shiny new future. I looked for signs along the way, just like Ashlad, I listened to advice and picked up strange things along the way that might be of use. Ashlad saw the potential in everything. The castle, symbolising his dreams, was bathed in a golden light. Gold is the purest metal known to man and symbolises the sun and the highest number we have, the number 9. That was my goal!

In numerology, this number stands for mediator and for completion. When I add up all the numbers of my own birthdate, I get the end number 9, which in numerology is my 'life path number'. One night I had a dream (Chapter 12: Dream nr 16: Time was 24:12) where the time was 24:12 and I was about to give birth to something. I knew what I was about to give birth to would *change everything*. I also knew I would have to let go of everything known to me. I was wondering if it was possible to avoid having to do go through with it, because I was scared to death of this delivery.

In the morning, I was lying in my bed with an inexplicable sense of fear. I started meditating and it slowly dawned on me it was all about the fear of giving birth to myself. In Norway, we associate December 24 with Christmas Eve, where we celebrate that humanity has been given a great gift. My dream is telling me I am afraid of giving birth to my gifts – my spiritual power. Heaven and Earth are to be united and balanced in me. I was dead scared of bringing forward the light in me, but somehow, I also knew it was the time.

Before I can receive the new life, I must let go of what has occupied this place for the most of my life. The science recognises our emotions have a mass. It is energy that occupies space. The emptiness that unavoidably is felt when we let go of the old and the new that is not yet born, often creates great fear. Fear of this emptiness, this stillness, can be overwhelming, but here is where the seed of light is found. In the stillness it will grow stronger – until I am ready to allow it to be born. In this process I am not supposed 'to do' anything but 'let Go and let God'. That was an ever-going struggle with my ego.

At this time, I had a dream (Chapter 12: Dream nr 17: I was in a basement) where I was in a basement looking for something to wear for an outing. I was going out into the forest to work on a project with a friend and colleague. He was waiting impatiently for me and this made me a bit unsettled. He was dressed in a warm check red work shirt and had a large and full backpack. He was well-equipped standing there on top of the stairs. I still had not found anything that seemed suitable. Suddenly I discovered my beautiful daughter June next to me. She walked up to a clothesline in the basement and pulled down a large and warm cape made from thick, pure white wool and was edged with a narrow golden band. "Mum, this is nice. You don't need anything else!" she told me. I knew that she was right and put it on and followed my colleague. I did not bring anything else. As we entered the forest, we only found dead trees. There was no green vegetation. I stopped and realised I was not supposed to go into this dying forest. Then I woke up.

My colleague and I had spent much time and resources to arrange a seminar we were about to conduct together in Oslo. We had put together a good outline and a binder with our marketing strategy. The dream told me clearly that this would lead us nowhere. I had everything needed as far as resources and protection, symbolised by my clean white and warm cape, but the forest was dead. Nothing would come of this collaboration. This turned out to be correct. No one signed up for the seminar. It had never happened to me before.

My intention was pure, but this was not the way my power was to be used. My colleague was well equipped for his next task. His backpack was full of knowledge and qualities that he was to use in another context. My own journey was to take me in a direction that was still below the horizon. I was led and supported to move on one day at a time, just listening.

I had several more dreams at this point. It seemed like 'the dreamer' in me was happy to finally be heard and wanted to show me more. In one dream (Chapter 12: Dream nr 18: A perfect house) I received confirmation that I was about to create new and positive thoughts about myself. The *light* inside was growing. In the dream I was walking around in an unknown neighbourhood looking for a new place to live. The houses were lovely and unique and creative like those you can find in parts of California. I was thinking I most likely could not afford something there, but still entered to check out one house that I really liked – just for the fun of it. A couple came forward to me. They were friendly and warm and showed me into their living room. It was as if I had designed and furnished it myself. It was open with a high ceiling. The walls were whitewashed and there were dark wooden beams in the ceiling framing certain sections of the room. The furniture was elegant and simple. I could have moved straight in. The garden was green and lush, and the kitchen was inviting and opened into the garden. I asked what they wanted for the house and expected it to be way out of my reach. When they answered 2,600,000 kroner, I thought with surprise this was exactly what I had! In the reality, I certainly did not have that amount of money, but the dream told me I had exactly what I needed. The dream also told me the place I wished to live was willing to receive me – when I was ready to give 'of myself'.

26 is my birthdate, and as mentioned before this number stands for healing power, creativity and cooperation. I just had to use my gifts and my story. All the zeroes emphasized the creative, intuitive and spiritual power available. The universe will support me if I am just willing to give of myself. The dream made me feel at ease and safe. I had nothing to fear – except for my own fear.

There is only one thing that makes a dream impossible to achieve: the fear of failure.

– Alberto Villoldo

I listened and sensed everything life offered, and sometimes I must discard some of the choices. We are given tests involving choices to help us become aware of what we really want. And then, of course, I get tested in a meditation setting I was involved in.

The meditation had started. It was participating in a guided meditation accompanied by beautiful music. I moved into the silence deep into the centre of my being where I got in touch with the *light*. I was pulled through different levels where the *light* changed colours as I moved through the levels. I felt I was getting filled up and become one with the *light*. Everything was peaceful and harmonious. The meditation slowly comes to an end and I returned with renewed strength and courage.

We are a welcoming little group who meet regularly to meditate together. The atmosphere was calm and peaceful as everyone slowly returned to the room. Then refreshments were served and for a short while all was well. But it did not take long before some on the team had the 'latest news' to share. It was about the scary conspiracies happening around the world.

Fear was slowly given power and the whole group was soon involved in a deep, intense conversation about everything scary and things that are 'worse than we can imagine'. I could sense the strength and peace that was to sustain me through my every day was slowly diminishing. I must consciously choose not to get into the fear energy. It is not that I do not know or want to know, but I must choose what I want to spend energy on. I love this little team but gave up after several efforts to stop this bad habit. Thought is energy and it creates and strengthens its own vibration. The choice is mine. I only want to protect and nourish the light growing inside of me now.

One day, I was sitting in deep meditation at home. I was using music played by Aborigines, the indigenous people of Australia, for inspiration. The music was strong and rhythmic. Suddenly, I was sitting outside in the dark by a campfire. I sat there quietly just being. To my surprise, a picture of Doris Day was put on my throat. This picture was very foreign in this setting. Surprised, I momentarily went out of my meditation and started analysing the vision. Personally, I connect Doris Day with a happy songbird with a nice energy. To be as 'nice' as Doris Day seemed not always to be the right. I had been able to remove the blockages in my breath and the power through my voice, but now I was reminded to use this newly acquired strength and speak my truth. The truth can sometimes be scary. The true strength within me was about to awaken.

One morning, I was not really sleeping but was not awake either when I saw a tall, very dark African man standing by the end of the bed. I got very scared, but as he just stood there calmly looking at me, I calmed down. He was a shaman with strong eyes. At first glance, he seemed incredibly scary, but then I realised he was a facet of myself. I studied him for a while and felt the fear was slowly letting go. I did recognise this power within me, like a primal force hiding there in my cell memories. The picture of my true power was slowly appearing. The power was both light and dark and I had to embrace it all.

Chapter 13
The Gate Breaks Open

Remember your thoughts are not original, brilliant or creative – your instincts, ideas and ability to dream are.

– Alberto Villoldo

To break through the limitations my ego had placed on my path I had to break down the wall of resistance I had put up. It was now about to give way. The light within grew stronger. I was ready to see my gifts and divine path.

Currently my dad was extremely ill. For a few years he had suffered from lupus. His condition had gotten far worse of late and was attacking vital organs. Somehow, I knew his time was soon ending. Then I dreamt (Chapter 13: Dream nr 19: In a forest with dad) I was in a forest with my dad. We were standing there under a high open night sky covered with stars. We built a small altar with little rocks placed around it like an altar rail. It seemed like a sacred moment. Dad wore his priest gown as he turned towards me and said, "Now, it's your turn." I understood it was my turn to give communion. I was not an ordained pastor, but it seemed like this was what ought to happen. I was in awe and deeply grateful to have been trusted with this task, but I did not really know what it entailed. Then I woke up.

The dream was both holy and symbolic to me. It was a sacred ritual where I understood I was shown my inner authority (priest) which gave me acceptance and recognition. The dream was an important confirmation that I was now my own authority. It was an acknowledgement of the mediator (sharing), this is also communicated in the number nine (my life number). Nine was also my dad's life number. At the time of my dream I could not see why we were standing outside in the nature. Much later, I received an explanation when I became a shaman apprentice. The shaman 'sees and heals' in cooperation with everything in nature. They know everything is sacred. This dream showed me I wished to be part of this magical world. I wanted to connect with the spirit in all the creation. It was all up to me…

Again, my awakening demanded several confrontations with my ego and the issues stopping me from moving on. My gifts and inheritance are kept safe in a treasure-chest inside my being. The ego is a strict protector, safeguarding the door to this place. It has 'protected' me all these years and resists the changes and every attempt to release my potential. That is, it's nature. Now, it is strongly challenged.

The planet Saturn in my birth-chart symbolises the guardian and the teacher of my shadow. It reveals the characteristics and roles my ego adopts to nourish, strengthen and protect its own existence. It shows me which shadow-sides I must master to liberate my hidden gifts – deep inside myself. In my birth-chart Saturn is in the sign of Libra. Everything has two sides, as does Libra. The shadow side or the challenge for Libra is to dear confrontations and make decisions. If I take the bull by the horns and challenge Saturn, the power and gift of Libra is liberated. These gifts are balance, harmony and beauty. My biggest challenge is also my greatest potential. The gift was trapped in my weakness – that was my fear! I was ready to confront it all now.

The symptoms show what unused power in me that is trying to wake me up to. In a dream (Chapter 13: Dream nr 20: The darkness was dens) I had now I was in a basement. It was pitch dark. I knew I had to pick up the courage to go into the next room. The darkness was dense and foreboding but I had no choice than to go in. I sensed someone was there and was scared – very scared. Slowly two tall beings stepped forward. They seemed *huge* and were completely covered in black hooded robes. Paralysed with fear, I stood there not able to move nor was I able to talk. Then they opened their robes and I saw a pulsating universe with a strong light within them. I was hit with the tremendous power and beauty of the vision as they communicate telepathically that I did not have to be afraid. They appeared to be two angels or seraphs, who had an important mission deep inside me. I woke up with greater self-esteem but also deeply shaken. Something inside me was exposed. My darkest place was hiding beautiful power!

The basement symbolises our subconscious, the unused and unowned power within. I had to go down there to meet my fear. The dream was showing me that what I always had been so afraid of is nothing to fear. The figures symbolised two sides of Saturn, that is my challenger and teacher. It challenges me to be conscious and responsible – and rewards me when I have learned to balance my power. Then true authority would be ready to take place in me.

Darkness contains no evil. It is neutral. It is our fear of the power that lies in darkness that causes pain. In darkness there is power to heal, like the rejuvenating sleep at night-time and the darkness of the soil nourishing the seed. The darkness holds a power and potency where all the colours are hiding. *Awareness is the light liberating the potential* (colours). When both dark and light cooperate, the power can be used to create something beautiful and new. The gate to my heart was slowly braking open – even if it creaks a bit.

Dad was on his deathbed. I had plenty of time and therefore was staying with him a lot. My father was to become an important part of the process I was going through at the time. He did not have the strength to talk, but still tried to sometimes. He looked at me and was able to mutter 'Why?' I knew intuitively he was asking me why I had not become 'who I really am'. I answered simply, "I didn't have the language." And then everything returned to silence. He understood and I knew I was now ready to express myself and who I am. No excuses.

Just before Dad died, I had a strange dream (Chapter 13: Dream nr 21: Confronting my fear). In my dream I was standing in a big courtyard with many people, including Dad. It was evening, and we were standing outside a big conference-centre admiring a dark and clear sky covered with stars. We saw some strange and beautiful constellations moving fast around the sky. The stars drew a dolphin standing up with his snout towards the west. There were also twelve more stars playing across the sky. Suddenly a big UFO came out of the sky and landed in front of us. A very tall being stepped off the UFO.

His body was a man's body but with the head of a ram with huge horns. I was very scared as I knew he came for me. The authority of this creature was so overwhelming that I could not escape. It was if it was representing a higher power. Dad walked between me and this scary creature. He was also afraid but also incredibly angry and wanted to protect me. He said he would go with this creature in my place. I asked Dad to simply accept this was my journey, and then with a pounding heart I went where I knew I had to go.

I woke up feeling shaken and empowered at the same time. In the Norwegian language, the name of the first sign I the Zodiac in English, is Aries (the Ram), is Vær. Translated into English would be the word 'Be' just simply to be triggers fear in us all and is as challenging as experiencing total emptiness or stillness. It takes great strength to simply be. Our surroundings will not accept this, nor will our built-in conditioning. The astrological sign Aries represents leadership, integrity, authority as well as intuitive strength and understanding. It has its physical seat at our third eye, the chakra between our eyebrows. The ram declares "I am". I have the planet Jupiter that representing luck, expansion and success in this star sign. *If I am myself, I will succeed.* Haven't I heard this before?

The UFO represents a higher form of awareness coming from outside – a higher consciousness. My desire to expand my consciousness demands me to let go of all what I know. I must leave my 'father's house' and protection and take charge of my own life. I must allow intuition (the third eye), my higher knowing, to guide me out of the old, collective thought patterns. I must follow my own authority. The starry sky represents guidance from above and challenges me to continuously 'read the signs'. The universe is our university.

The dolphin that the stars drew in the sky, symbolises childlike play, joy and unconditional love. It is to teach me how to breathe freely and flow with the pulse of the universe without fear. The nose pointed towards the West tells me I had to dare to follow my heart and go to America. This dream was growing stronger.

Here I was again receiving a couple of nudges. As my inner sun was growing stronger, this power was pulling me toward the 'sunny place' in the physical world. But I must step back at times, for the universe to be able to put in place the necessary pieces of the puzzle. I must rest in the stillness, to simply be and trust. This is difficult for the ego who wants to control, act and direct. Time and again I must be convinced by my heart before accepting who I am—whom I now more often meet in the stillness—in being-ness. Franz Kafka says, "You do not need to leave your room. Remain sitting at your table and listen. Do not even listen, simply wait, be quiet, still and solitary. The world will freely offer itself to you to be unmasked, it has no choice, it will roll in ecstasy at your feet."

Your intent is for the future, but your attention is in the present. As long as your attention is in the present, then your intent will manifest, because the future is created in the present.

– Deepak Chopra

Priests in Norway have an unclarified relationship with healers, to say the least. Dad therefore had a problem with calling me a healer or spiritual counsellor. I was presented as an art therapist, and this was of course not incorrect. Privately we agreed I could be called a Christian mystic. Toward the end, when Dad did not have the strength to talk, I would come and sit quietly with him in the Hospital. Once a nurse entered the room. Dad caught her attention with a small gesture, gathered strength and said to her, "This is my daughter Gro. She is a healer."

He looked at me and whispered, "Honour to whom honour is due that's what you are Gro." This is the greatest gift I have received next to the gift of life and my children who 'chose' me to be their mother. It helped me to open the door to the great *light* within.

I started receiving more confirmations about who I am. It seemed the universe was out to convince me now. I was attending a healing seminar. We were paired up to lead each other on an inner journey. My partner was Ingrid, a beautiful and strong person. I was to lie down on the bench first and Ingrid was to guide me into a deep meditation. It did not take long before I was led far down into the quiet centre of my being. When I confirmed I was there, Ingrid asked me to open a door to the left. As I opened it, I was blinded by the light coming at me. Inside the room was an overwhelmingly beautiful and strong light being. Ingrid asked me gently to walk into this room. I was paralysed with reverence and the beauty of the dazzling light. Ingrid got no response when she asked me what was happening. After a little while, she became anxious because it seemed like I was completely gone, so she called out my name several times. I heard someone calling my name far away but could not answer. I was too overwhelmed. After a small eternity I was able to mutter 'yes', but I felt I said 'yes' to the light being. I came to understand the *light* was an aspect of myself and if I answered 'yes' to this, I had to accept myself and my name. This is what was so difficult, to accept Gro. My name suddenly became very real to me. It seemed like I had not been conscious of my name or who I was up until this moment. The day after the seminar, I met a good friend and colleague. We were having a cup of coffee and talking about what we had experienced in our lives recently. When I told him of what happened the day before, he looked at me in wonder and asked, "Did you realise yesterday was your name day?" I had no idea and newer bothered to learn about that. Interesting, I had accepted my name on my name day!

Life continued – but now into a bigger and more magical universe. I had accepted my name and seen my inner power. Now, I was ready to receive this power lying dormant within. I was resting on a bench having acupuncture done by a beautiful, strong woman in Norway. It was a gift from a friend. As she placed the needles the woman asked gently if she could do some healing work while we were waiting for the effect of the needles. I gratefully accepted. I felt so blessed. She led me into a deep and peaceful relaxation exercise. Suddenly, I felt like I became a gorilla! I was filled with a big, strong, peaceful and good-natured gorilla with clear turquoise eyes. I could feel its power throughout my body and all the way out into my fingertips. With my eyes closed and smiling, I mentioned this to the healer. She apologised shockingly, but I calmed her down and said I could feel it was a good force settling in me.

I really did not understand the meaning of this symbol at the time. Little is written about the symbol of gorillas to use for dream interpretation. Then I found the website www.whats/your/sign.com: The gorilla seems scary because it is so big and seemingly aggressive, but really it is the most docile of all monkeys. The gorilla is described as noble with great intelligence and integrity. He is a loyal creature, responsible and with strong leadership abilities and a very social and caring animal, also symbolising mobility and playfulness.

The turquoise eyes showed my soul's purpose regarding this power. The eyes are the window of the soul, and the light in his eyes was turquoise symbolising healing. I read if a gorilla shows up in a dream, it is a sign to lift your head and recognise your own noble nature, and to act with integrity. I must dare to appear scary if that is what is needed. Two years later, in Mexico, I was strangely to be reminded of this insight by an Indian Shaman.

Not long after this experience I was invited to join a group who would be visited by Iliuka, an old highly advanced soul who is channelled by the Norwegian medium and shaman Leif Havik. When it was my time to receive an answer to a question I had prepared, I asked what I was to do with the sorrow I was carrying. "It's not the sorrow, *but the sun inside that you are withholding,*" he said. Finally, I received a confirmation and reminder of something that I already knew. It is the light that I am holding back that is causing me to become depressed and ill. "Just throw rocks…" Iliuka said. He recognised I needed an outlet for the frustration that was blocking the sun in me.

A couple of weeks later, on a beautiful autumn day my friend Liv and I were on our way to take a mountain hike. We wanted to use our voices freely and powerfully, so we agreed to join up and go to a place where we could be out in nature on our own. I had also decided I wanted to 'throw rocks'. After a four-hour drive and enjoying a good cup of coffee we started on our hike. The scenery was overwhelmingly beautiful. I picked up a rock, breathed deeply and blew all my sorrow and perceived pain inside into the rock. With my inner eye I saw the rock filled with blood. Then I asked mother earth to take it all and threw the rock at another large rock – and it cracked. I felt emptied out. I closed my eyes as I was leaning my back up against a big rock and felt a strong power rise from inside.

Suddenly from deep within I started a powerful chant. It seemed like an old and strong voice of a shaman carried through me and across the highlands. I allowed the power to fill me and my voice to take wings and fly unrestrained. While I was still chanting, Liv drew my attention to a herd of hundreds of reindeer thundering right towards us. I knew from deep inside that I had called on them. Stunned, I stopped chanting, and at that very moment the whole herd stopped abruptly. For a long second, they stood there quietly looking at us before the whole herd suddenly turned to the left and continued their journey.

These abilities that are in all of us have been lying dormant through many generations and are now shaking us awake. When my voice is true and flows powerfully without fear, I can call on and communicate with nature in a simple and powerful way. The integrity of my voice was received by the nature. The gate between heaven and earth in me, between my heart and mind and between me and the nature is opening. I am slowly stepping forward.

Chapter 14
One Step Back

Emotions reflect intentions. Therefore, awareness of emotions leads to awareness of intentions.

– Gary Zukav

The gate was now opening but I did not really dare to go through it all the way. I had arrived at a point where I had to totally empty my boat. Everything I had learned and understood to this point asked this of me before I could step out into my own light. I experienced the darkness before dawn and again fear got a hold of me. It was as if I had to go through some type of dying process before I could receive new life. I was so close to something big that scared me into stepping back for a short while.

My body needed warmth and sunshine. I had to acknowledge my body and soul did not thrive here in Norway. I wanted out but something inside me tried to calm me down and help me to have trust in the process. The time had not yet come I was told in a dream (Chapter 14: Dream nr 22: I was on a still going raft) where I was sitting on a raft with my youngest son at the helm. We were quietly flowing through dense fog in a slow-moving calm river. Around us was a mangrove forest. It was mystical and beautiful, with vegetation and branches leaning over the river. I was unsettled we did not move faster, but my son asked me to calm down. "Be completely quiet, Mum," he said. Then I woke up.

I knew it was okay that I had to be so still although it almost felt like I was taking a few steps backwards. I did not have to be ashamed or criticise myself because this was happening. Moments like this are natural and necessary for a seeker. I am moving through an unknown foggy emotional landscape and must take it one step at a time. In this dream, the water illustrates my emotional landscape. My son, the active aspect of myself in the dream, knew there was a time and place for everything. I just had to let go and be. It truly felt like I was dying, but I had to admit it was simply the ego losing control.

Self-sabotage is not a stranger to me, and it strikes every time I am about to see the greatness inside. The ego knows the stillness is the doorway to who I am – and dare not allow me to meet the power living there. That is why the stillness was so important but also so threatening at this point.

The great French thinker and mathematician Blaise Pascal, writes in his book Pensées, 'All of humanity's problems stem from man's inability to sit quietly in a room alone.'

During moments of weakness, I comforted myself with the thought that even great masters had fought this battle. Stillness seems to be one of the most difficult challenge we as humans are faced with. The place where seemingly nothing happens, and we believe that our lives will fall apart. We seem to forget changes are happening in the depth of the silence – in the cocoon.

It is 'The dark night of the soul' that the Spanish mystic San Juan de la Cruz so famously write about.

Life appears to be like a beautiful tapestry where many backstitches are needed to create the right depiction. "Take one stitch at a time, Gro!" my departed father told me through a channel in Norway. I realised patience was not a virtue I possessed yet and neither did my father. It was a paradox that he was the one pointing this out. Was he taking responsibility for transmitting this restless pattern on to me maybe? I smiled. *You are right,* I thought!

Then I dreamt (Chapter 14: Dream nr 23: Helping Mum to move) I was helping Mum to move. We were almost done but the last stage was going awfully slow and I was getting exasperated. Mum would immerse herself in old memories and was also very meticulous with the packing. Everything was moving painfully slow. I had to ask the young girls moving into our place to wait another 15 minutes. It seemed important to give Mum the time she needed, but I was still restless. I could sense the young people's anticipation and tried to be as optimistic as possible. While waiting I went into the kitchen. It showed the pipes in the kitchen were clogged with a white dough. This also had to get fixed before the girls could move in, I thought. If I had not been forced to wait, I would not have discovered this problem. I knew the 15 minutes would not be enough to get the job done. Again, I had committed to something I could not keep, just to be nice.

As I woke up that morning, I realised I had more to straighten out before moving on. Mum is incredibly careful and patient. Here she is showing me I must accept the time it takes to get something done properly. I realis I keep pushing myself and do not give myself enough time. The young people represent an aspect of me that was still immature and restless. They mirrored what I still feared from my surroundings. I had to strengthen and live in integrity, as my inner 'gorilla' wanted. I must be true to myself.

I realised the white dough showed me I had eaten refined foods that did not give any nourishment. I must choose the 'nourishment' that will be beneficial and get rid of everything else. The kitchen symbolises the heart. I wanted my time and space for my process – with no excuses.

Then I had another dream that reinforced the message in the previous one. In my dream (Chapter 14: Dream nr 24: Picked up by an UFO) it was night-time, and I was driving a car on a deserted road towards a city. A huge UFO descended from the night sky and suddenly I was in it. I was asked to sit down on a small white couch. I could not see anything else in the very white surroundings. A woman dressed in all white and with dark hair sat down beside me to the left. Everything looked 'normal' in my corner. I had the feeling everything was arranged in this way to help me feel safe and gain confidence in her. The woman told me telepathically, I was intolerant to the foods I was eating. Then after pausing she said I also was intolerant to the water I was drinking. I woke up thinking, what do I do now?

Just for the record, I was not much into UFO's and did not really look up much information on that subject nor did I attend any such interest groups. That is why I was so surprised to have these dreams of UFO's that symbolise a higher consciousness and awareness.

It was obvious the dream warned me about things I was taking in. I felt I was starting to get allergic to everything around me. Not just food and drink, but also the mental and emotional 'nourishment'. I could not digest much of it. Several things were weakening me, both physically as well as mentally. Water, symbolising feelings, showed I was sensitive towards the many unbalanced feelings around me – as well as inside of me. We tell each other stories and news that are not uplifting and use each other as 'trash cans' without really understanding what is happening. We really do not understand we are part of everything – and therefore also co-creators of everything. Obviously, I had to be more conscious in all my choices. My inner gorilla needed to be consulted.

There is so much to learn. Some tell me time is an illusion. When I do not really understand what is happening, I simply need to slow down, like my son reminded me of in the dream where we were floating together (Chapter 14: Dream nr 22: I was on a still going raft). Our individual need for *time* and space to heal is not the focus of self-help seminars or books. The healing-process takes time. Time is money, which again often pushes us into be miserable.

I had to stop pushing myself or allow others to push me. I had to simply breathe deeply and accept the time it would take to give birth to me. I had to create the needed distance from my emotions and float freely and quietly while simply listening and looking up towards the sky – to the stars.

If I am a part of the universe, then it is not strange the universe with all its synchronicity also reflects my inner universe. Macro cosmos mirrors mini cosmos and reversely. My inner network of energy fields has its blueprint in the outer universe. There is mutual mirroring which also has mutual impact. We live in this energetic interaction between the outer and inner world, where everything influences all. The Hungarian author and spiritual teacher Elisabeth Haich say, "Each star sign describes a facet of God's face and being." We carry a part of the nature of God within. We are creators. My ego doesn't want me to see and acknowledge this.

Logic will get you from A to B. Imagination will take you everywhere.
– Albert Einstein

My ego fears dying and calls itself 'reasonable', as it tries to hold me back. My rational mind was obviously not yet able to let go and let the old die. I had a peek into the Promised Land but maybe did not think I deserved entering it just yet – or maybe I was just imagining all this?

Many great mathematicians, scientists and philosophers have admitted that all innovation starts with a fantasy, a dream. 'You are gifted with an incredible imagination!' was an observation from a well-renowned American intuitive. "You have been given an incredible imagination, but you are getting in your own way," he added. My analytical mind often blocked the way for my imagination. I was my own worst enemy. Thought and heart must start up a conversation before I can manoeuvre my life into calmer seas.

At this point, I also experienced being told by a well-meaning person that maybe now was a good time to let go of my dream and stop believing in it! I felt myself fading and lost my footing, as if someone gave me a fatal wound. I breathed in deeply and changed the topic. I realised this person might have given up her own dream. It is easy to project your own issues onto others. At the same time, my doctor suggested maybe it was time to start on some medication – some antidepressant. I was speechless.

Don Miguel Ruiz writes in his book 'The Mastery of Love' about the reason of misusing drugs often is connected to low self-acceptance. One's own inner critic becomes so loud one feels the need to make oneself insensible to be able to be with oneself. I had observed the misuse of medication in my close circle. I had also observed what damage this 'medication' has done to the ability of self-healing. Drugs remove our willpower.

I know the pain I experience is the only thing that can tell me what I feel and what is needed to heal. Am I supposed to drug down the only thing that can enlighten and guide me in the healing process? When will I then be able to become who I am, well, healed, free and a creative human being?

You do not attract what you want. You attract what you are.

– Wayne Dyer

Dr Wayne Dyer, one of our time's great spiritual teacher, stresses all thoughts and feelings that do not do us good, resists the source within, or if you will, the God image in all of us. Alberto Villoldo expressed it as follows, "Non-judgment leads to non-illness." I must stop judging myself. My inner critic would pop up regularly, but now I did not listen to it in the same way as I used to. Something was moving on inside me.

One night I dreamt (Chapter 14: Dream nr 25: Advice from my son) I asked a friend, who most likely also had a strong inner critic, what to do. Before she had the time to answer my oldest, wise son appeared beside me and said in a friendly manner, "It's all about seeing what you think, because this leads to attitudes which in turn lead to action, Mum."

I smiled at him proud and in awe. I said, "That's exactly what we are working towards, my son!" I woke up and understood I already know what to do, but I must be more present in my thinking. I realised the need I had to be alone and secluded had to do with a deep longing to be close to myself, to be in my own space – on my own terms. I wanted to hear myself.

In this quiet space, the optimism can grow without getting challenged or uprooted during this tender stage before the roots have attached. Something beautiful was about to grow strong. I did not phone anyone, nor write. It was my own quiet journey. After a while I started to really enjoy this quiet space. I was nourished by the stillness when I allowed myself to simply rest in it. I was strengthened and slowly started to enjoy living. This is not the normal way of measuring 'doing well'. I see the fear of being alone is projected when someone is concerned about me, but I do not expect to be understood. Finally, I have stopped caring so much about this. I grow and heal in the stillness and healing empty space.

I am my own best friend and meditation is my self-medication. I found the quietest spot inside and settled down and stayed there like a bear in hibernation. I did this till finally spring arrived in my mind.

Chapter 15
The All and I

Just like a sunbeam cannot separate itself from the sun, and a wave can't separate itself from the ocean, we can't separate ourselves from one another. We are all part of a vast sea of love, one indivisible divine mind.

— Marianne Williamson

In the stillness of my inward journey I rediscovered hidden and forgotten aspect of myself. Important pieces to the puzzle fell into place. A dawning trust and believing that I truly was a part of the whole, helped me to accept the messages.

Pictures from my childhood appeared and reminded me of who I really am, deep inside. It shed light upon a forgotten and hidden memory; I was about 12 years' old standing outside the boarding school in Ngaoundere. It was Sunday, the quietest day of the week. Most of the others were on outings while my siblings and I were among the few left, seemingly forgotten and invisible to the adults.

I held a straw and allowed my thoughts to wander. Suddenly, I felt I was becoming smaller and smaller. I feared I would disappear when noticing I was as small as an insect on the straw in my hand. At the same time, all distances around me grew so large I felt that I might as well have been the only one in the universe. Then suddenly, I started growing. I grew and grew and finally was so huge that it was beyond description. I filled up the universe. It was wonderful, but baffling – and scary. I figured I best be quiet about this strange and mystical experience.

One day, 40 years later, I sat in the office of therapist and healer Kaja Finne. It had been a long time since I last visited her. We talked about everything and nothing when she suddenly looked at me thoughtfully asking me to go within to the stillness inside and become as small as possible. I did what I was told and suddenly the memory awakened when I as a child experienced being as small as an insect and next growing so large that I filled all the universe. Kaia intuitively followed my process. When she asked me to become as large as possible, she could 'see' what was happening and said, "Now, you are ready." I knew it to be true.

Intuition is a spiritual faculty and does not explain, but simply points the way.

– Florence S. Shinn

As the story goes, a native Indian enters a room, and first takes in the energy of the place before he greets each person. This way, he already knows quite a bit about each person in the room. A joint energy is created, and we become part of it whether we know it or not. Everything and everyone has influence.

I realised I do not need to be tossed around in a boat out in the ocean, helplessly in the waves. What if I simply recognise that I am part of the great big ocean and not separate from it? If I am part of the ocean, I am no longer the victim tossing about aimlessly but carried by the waves. I am continually reminded to 'go with the flow'. If I become one with the elements and energy around me, I am no longer just part of the problem, but also part of the solution. If I work with everything, I am also supported by everything.

I cannot change and control anything outside of myself, only what is inside. The only thing I have power to change is my own reaction. If I relax, my surroundings will be affected. Emotions are waves of energy in motion. I am therefore a co-creator of my surroundings and environment.

If I were *not* creating fear or doubt, things simply would work themselves out. Fear is an energy creating resistance. I had to trust the waves. My growing ability to trust was now confirmed through an everyday happening. I jumped on a bus going to the centre of town and did not register the number of the bus. This central station was large with many buses all going into centre of Oslo. After spending several hours in town, I noticed my credit card was gone. I had no idea where it could be and prayed it would be protected and safe. I imagined a bubble of light around the card and visualised it was returned to me. Through experience I now knew worry and fear never created good solutions. I therefore chose to stay calm and trust everything would work out simply fine. When I returned home later in the day, I asked the bus driver if he could please phone the head office and ask if anyone had turned in a credit card that day. "Could it be this one?" he asked and gave me my card. It turned out to be the same bus driver that I had travelled with earlier in the day. "I was just going off duty," he said. The chances of this happening seemed ridiculously small. Magical moments are created when we choose to be open to it. We are really connected to 'It All'.

All my strange experiences and magical moments felt important and needed to be shared, I thought. The idea of writing a book had started to take shape after having an exceptional dream.

To write a book when you have only learned Norwegian as an adult is quite ambitious. But then I remembered what my teacher in arts in high school told me. He told me I was good at drawing but did not have colour perception. A few years later I was a painter and was teaching in the subject, and I was even told I was good in it – and gifted.

In this dream (Chapter 15: Dream nr 26: By an old stairway), I was standing in a basement by an old stairway. The stairway and the railing were made from old wood. Two older women stood there, and both pointed at a small yellow pencil lying on the floor in front of my feet. Telepathically, they instructed me to pick it up and use it. It was a short little stub, only about an inch. Then they handed me a curled-up piece of paper and communicated I should start using it. They both had authoritative energy and it seemed they were 'wise women' and strong healers. In the dream, I did not recognize neither of them. One had fair hair and was called Astrid. The other had dark hair and was called Ragnhild.

I woke up a bit confused and wondered who these women were and what this dream could mean. As mentioned, writing was not my forte. But the desire to share and convey my experiences was great. The small pencil stub was a clear illustration of the 'small tool' or 'small ability' I had regarding writing. The basement represents the subconscious and those two women were both aspects of my feminine heritage and power. With time I learned Astrid was my deceased grandmother, who I never really learned to know well. I only knew she was a good person with a big heart. I remember Astrid having white hair. Ragnhild showed up to be my father's aunt who I never met. My father admitted Ragnhild had some unusual gifts. She had dark hair and was strong and intuitive. What they both communicated to me seemed important. I got started right away. I felt I could trust them and knew they would help me.

Not long after I had another dream (Chapter 15: Dream nr 27: A black notebook) confirming the above. I dreamt about a black notebook which reminded me of a journal I had at that time. In the dream I was already halfway through writing it. We were many people sitting around a long dinner table, decorated for a party. The black book was lying on a large, beautiful white plate in front of me. A dark-haired charming Spanish man had put it before me. I was his dinner partner and it was an official gala dinner. He picked up the book and started reading from it aloud. It was about a travel adventure. Suddenly the story turned into a game board, unfolding on the table in front of us, like a fairytale setting. On the board was a picture of a landscape with woods and fields and a yellow path winding through the landscape. Small figures also popped up on the board. They were fun looking. It looked very humorous.

Then I found a pile of liquorice strings on my plate and some colourful round liquorice candy. I was mesmerised. My dinner partner seemed quite reserved in the beginning but with time showed up to be a warm and wise person, although his teeth were filed pointedly and sharp. He was pleasantly surprised about my positive response when he stood up and read from my book with enthusiasm and warmth. I was touched and happy and woke up with a good feeling.

The dream told me to convey my strange experiences and the playful, humoristic and creative dream travels into my book, I thought. Yellow symbolises knowledge, joy and communication. This colour permeated the whole landscape, like a road or thread and showed up in the eyes of the little creatures as sparks of life and joy. A table indicates sharing. The candies on the plate next to the book, were perhaps sweet rewards? I interpreted the liquorice strings to be threads of joy and excitement from my journeys. All was meant to be shared.

The astrological sign of Spain is the Sagittarius. An optimistic, freedom-loving, philosophical sign that also and always is travelling – looking for the truth. Sagittarius is centrally located twice in my own astrological birth-chart and therefore know I have the gift of these energies. The Spanish man was an aspect of my desire for action, communication and adventure. His sharp teeth show I need to 'sharpen my pen' and not be afraid of expressing myself clearly and honestly. The official public gathering showed I should not be afraid to give of myself. The dream settled in the back of my consciousness. It was all strangely connected, but my book had to wait. I was not ready.

Dreams do not have to be understood right away, but with time they will perhaps show what the message is all about. The time gives us perspective and makes it easier to understand what was conveyed to us. If we do not understand everything in a dream, we can simply accept the essence of what the dream seems to express and realise the process continues in the subconscious. The process happens in the quiet, secluded space. Everything is chewed, broken down and processed in this cocoon of silence. The information regarding who I really am is all there and helps me recode my life. Everything is changing. Was it all only growing pains?

I was now 57 years old and my health was still a big challenge, but my spirit was willing to finish the race. I knew my spirit and body could communicate and work together now. But the deeper I went into my inner landscape the more aggressively the body responded, as the ego resisted the disclosure. I was getting closer – and the ego reacted panicky.

The specialist treating me recognised the strong psoriasis symptoms had to be psychosomatic. Finally, I thought and told her I knew I was the only one who could heal me. The professor looked at me pensively and quietly said, "You are a wise woman." I had told her I was using meditation and self-discovering as tools to heal.

As the light gets stronger the shadow also gets stronger – or clearer. I knew I could take advantage of this. I was willing to confront the deepest fear in me. Now, I dreamt (Chapter 15: Dream nr 28: Magic powers) I was with my ex-husband and some friends at a company party. I was dressed up and although I really did not like these events still was prepared to join in. As we stepped into the venue, I was approached by a woman with evident dark, magical powers. She knew I had 'seen' her, and she was exposed. "You are holy," she whispered. I did not like her tone of voice and wanted to leave. I could feel I did not belong in this environment, so I decided to leave the party.

On my way out, three people were lined up on the left side. They did not think anyone could see them and thought they were invisible to common people. But I saw them. I saw they had strong powers which they used negatively. One woman had two pairs of eyes and another talked with two voices. The last one was a male with ginger hair and strong bluish-grey eyes. He appeared to be nice, friendly and charming but I knew he was misusing his powers and using his eyes to give him insight and control. To make sure he could not continue hurting others with this power, I had to poke my fingers into his eyes. I 'neutralised' all the three dark magicians before leaving. As I stepped outside, I heard a woman I knew cry for help. She was in another building and was fighting with a demon. I knew I would not be able to save her in time and simply had to acknowledge the fact I could not help everyone. Finally, I was out in the sunshine! I breathed in the wonderfully fresh air and felt so free. Then my mother appeared as a younger version of herself. She had on a pair of red, smart shorts and was skating on a red skateboard. She laughed and enjoyed mastering this new balancing act. I was impressed and happy for her. At this point, I woke up, surprised and strangely inspired.

The dream could have seemed both scary and confusing, but I knew it simply was telling me I now was ready to use my powers and gifts – to do good. I am again reminded that my greatest fear is of acknowledging my power and greatness. We live in a collective field where many energies are present and can influence us. This includes the dark collective history we share. I no longer feared these energies in myself or others. The fact that others could not see the negative energies in the room, is possibly because the shadow sides of many of the public are not acknowledged or admitted. *What you do not believe you are not able to see*. I was now able to see the shadow side, and both conquer and defuse them, because I had acknowledged my own power, and worked on my own shadow. The dream also reminded me I was not responsible to save everyone. I was free to go out and play.

My mum is a Gemini, an astrological sign that illustrates our potential to develop playfulness, curiosity and communicative abilities. The time had come for me to better balance the playfulness and seriousness. The skateboard illustrates balance and play. The red pair of shorts expresses action and freedom, joy and playfulness. I am about to learn an important lesson of balancing all aspects and strengths in my life – through the heart. In the dream, I took a firm stand regarding the fear of negative powers – both my own and others', and the reward was freedom, sunshine and play. The place I left was a collective thought-energy that had made me ill.

I not only have knowledge but also gifts that go far beyond what I previously realised. The magician in me slowly gets more acceptance and attention. What you focus on also is given more energy! What receives energy gains strength and grows! Gifts and knowledge are united, the creator and the thinker, the feminine and the masculine. I am growing.

One day, I was taking a stroll down a forest path. I enjoyed everything around me, the sights, the sounds and the smells. Finally, I had regained trust in the Norwegian environment and knew it was safe. I studied the grass, flowers and leaves and suddenly discovered some straws with black buds. They were so black that I did not really know if I liked them. They were almost scary I thought and suddenly I realised they were all over the place. I became conscious of my thoughts and quickly decided to turn my attention towards something else. I wanted to look for shiny rocks on the path, I thought. Suddenly it was as if all the rocks were shining and sparkling, to the point that I was almost dazzled. It showed me it was all about choices. My earlier fear of the Norwegian woods was now all gone. I could choose my way of seeing things. How powerful we are!

I did not want to delay anything now and felt ready to take the next step. I was reminded of the quote by Dorothy Bernard; Courage is fear that has said its prayers. So, it is all right that I was a bit fearful. But I must try! I could not allow fear to paralyse me. Courage comes from the source within which is stronger than my outer circumstances. When I acknowledge I am stronger than my problems I will receive the needed courage to overcome anything. Courage is the ability to meet what you imagine, even if it seems too large, strong or beautiful to be true.

Our deepest fear is not that we are inadequate. Our deepest fear is that we are powerful beyond measure. It is our light, not our darkness that most frightens us.

– Marianne Williamson

It scares me a bit that I am responsible for the great power I have discovered. Then I was reminded of what the channelled soul Iluka told me. *It is not the sorrow that weighs you down but the Sun that I have disallowed.* I must dare to shine reassured that I am protected and supported.

The Sun is my Power.

Of course, a challenge appeared now for my growth. A good friend popped by one day. She was experiencing anxiety attacks at night she explained. I told her she could *choose* to not accept these energies. She could simply stop accepting them, if she wanted to, I said. She could stop focusing on them by protecting herself and surrounding herself with light. The troll bursts when exposed to the light. It is so easy, but oh so difficult still.

The following night, right before drifting off to sleep, my whole bedroom was filled with dark shadow energy. The air was heavy, and it felt like it was taking all the oxygen in the room. I was overwhelmed with terrible anxiety like I had never experienced before. Then suddenly I remembered what I had advised my friend to do earlier that day and started the experiment: I closed my eyes and breathed in the light from a star I knew was right above my head. I had to really work hard on my breathing to let go of the fear and allow the light to enter. With every breath I took the power of the light got stronger. I allowed it to fill me up completely. I continued to breathe in light and slowly the whole room also was filled with light. After some time, there was no more room for the dark energies in or around me. As with the stroke of a magic wand I was filled with peace and my bedroom was again a nice and peaceful place to be.

Everything can be found inside of me because I am a part of everything. But I am reminded I only get what I am willing to receive. In my dreams I am shown everything I am not conscious of through symbols and illustrations from the collective treasure chest.

Here we can learn about archetypes: ancient symbols illustrating fundamental human traits and instincts and showing people or creatures from mythology and history that are humanity's cultural heritage. These are impersonal symbols showing deep patterns that we all share. We have all of nature and all these stories inside of us: inside of us:

-I am the lioness who stands proudly with authority, protecting and providing for her children and herself.

-I am the snake who has both the power to heal and to kill. It lies coiled at the base of the spine, ready to rise to its potential power. Its power is also psychic strength and clairvoyance.

-I am the jaguar who importantly has the power and the will to protect the heart. It sees and hears what others cannot and proceeds with true integrity and strength.

-I am the hummingbird who enjoys the nectar from the most beautiful flowers, drinking in the beauty of its surroundings. It is free to move in any direction on any level, a messenger between heaven and earth.

-I am the eagle, flying high above everything, experiencing the overview. It sees life in perspective and rest on the strong wings of intuition. It is holy and free and help our spirit to return home.

-I am the ant, busily and tirelessly fulfilling its role in the collective.

-I am the beaver who patiently rebuilding what the emotional river has torn down after a rainfall.

-I am the bear, resting in his cave without excuses or explanations. He simply does what he needs to do and rests in his strength.

-I am the wild boar, who confronts its surroundings if challenged.

-I am the lizard, sitting alert taking its place in the sun, warming its body on the heat-lamp of our universe. It does what its body tells it to do. It rests, feels the vibration of the earth, trusting its instinct.

I am everything and one with it all.

Everything existing in the Cosmos finds its reflection in my micro-Cosmos, in my inner Dreamland. The sun reflects the fire within; the moon the waters of my emotions. The earth reflects my body, the air in my breath and the spirit in the spark of life and joy in my heart.

Chapter 16
From Chaos to Cosmos

Fight for your Dreams and your Dreams will fight for you.

– Paulo Coelho

As an artist I know being in a creative process demands not fearing chaos. to be in a creative process. Brainstorming is the process where we start throwing out any ideas or associations we might have. Knowledge and common sense are thrown into the equation later. The inspiration must flow freely, unconditionally and with enthusiasm during the beginning stages. *The heart chooses, and the mind executes.* I had now learned: what I envisioned I create.

Something was starting to take form within me. I had allowed chaotic thoughts and experiences to be aired out and shone light on them, and slowly I could see a connection that made sense. I had been honest with myself while taking a stroll through my shadowland looking for myself and my dream. At this moment, I had a dream (Chapter 16: Dream nr 29: After a very long walk) showing I had walked extremely far all by myself. I had only had a half hour break with a bite to eat but that was several days ago. There was no more food and I was very tired. After having walked day and night through rough terrain I found myself next morning suddenly overlooking a beautiful, open green and lush landscape. Not far away, I could spot a small town with nice white houses shining along the shore. I was overjoyed to finally have arrived but also bewildered and proud that I had really seen this through despite all the difficulty I had encountered along the way. I had often felt very alone and scared struggling all night through forests and thickets. At times, I could not see a thing as I was walking ahead in the night-time in trust. At last, I had arrived safe and sound! I was ever so relieved.

I had been taking the journey trusting my heart and providence. The dream confirmed I had made the right choices through my process. Despite feeling I did not have enough food, strength or courage, I learned; *I did have everything I needed*. I just had to take one step at a time and endure. The long walk in the dark was illustrating much of the journey had been on an unconscious level. I had been willing to follow all the signs and symbols encountered on the way and finally I realized I do have the willpower, strength and ability to succeed. I now can live it!

My wish to have a longer stay in California was closer to my view, but still I could not see how that would happen. The sunshine, warmth and the people there seemed just what I needed. Was I ready for a serious choice? Would I really have to sell my apartment to make it happen? Not many would support me in this decision I thought. But I could not really afford my flat anyway. At this point, I had a dream (Chapter 16: Dream nr 30: A dark stormy ocean) where I was standing on the West coast of Norway overlooking a dark, stormy ocean. The waves hitting the shore were huge and threatening and the sky was dark and foreboding. I had decided to leave on a big ship that was now wrestling in the surf. I wanted to cross the ocean and go to America but was warned by the people around me. I still decided to go. As soon as I had this thought, I was on board the ship and everything went well.

What people feared was an illusion.

The dream supported me in my decision to leave. I should not let mine or others' fears affect me even if the situation seems impossible. The dark sky illustrates fear-based thoughts. The ocean is the symbol for the collective emotions which in this case were chaotic, out of balance or rebellious. I kept my vision and gave it more focus and energy. Although I was a bit unsettled, something still told me everything would be okay.

My visions were now lighter and more optimistic. I allowed myself to dream big. Then I dreamt (Chapter 16: Dream nr 31: A white shopping Centre) I was standing on the second floor of a white and lovely shopping centre with a large open midpoint. A beautiful wide staircase was winding from the upper level to the lower level of the mall. I was standing at the top and holding on to the railing while stretching towards a white shiny crystal chandelier hanging from the ceiling in the centre of the room. While holding on to the chandelier, I slid or floated down the railing to the first floor. The chandelier kind of moved with me down the stairs. It obviously could be pulled wherever I wanted. It appeared to be a new feature and offer at the centre, but people did not really understand what to use it for. I was acknowledged for showing how this light could be used and people started using it. I was incredibly happy when I woke up.

I think the dream was about what I realise I have to offer that is my own light. It is a gift everyone has, and many are starting to discover. The centre is a symbol of a collective level where everything is available regarding pure knowledge (light). I realize everything here in the centre has pure intention. The chandelier symbolize enlightenment. The Staircases represent the level of development in us. There is no effort in this, only pure and simple joy. Life is supposed to be easy to live and can be if we only liberate ourselves from all the limitations – which are fear-based thoughts. I bring along the chandelier, God's light or my higher consciousness through all the levels in me to cast light on and heal everything. I finally understand I have a wise, beautiful and reliable inner voice and beautiful inner self.

Have a mind that is open to everything and attached to nothing.
– Dr Wayne Dyer

I once learned how to interpret aura pictures. It seemed I had a gift along these lines. One day I was to interpret the aura of a person sitting in front of me. I did not know anything about him, and I did not know he was a doctor till I had interpreted his picture. The green heart chakra was overexposed. I explained there was a great leakage in his heart energy. I told him he was giving too much. His eyes welled up with tears and then he told me he was a medical doctor and explained about his hopeless working environment at the hospital where he worked. Since he worked with a holistic approach to illness at one of our large hospitals in Oslo, he was overrun by patients who only wanted him to attend to them. He did not know what to do about it and had a hard time saying no. The other doctors at this hospital did not want to work the way he did, therefore He felt alone in his responsibility for all the patients. I told him the only thing he could do both to help himself and others was to learn to say 'no'. I explained it was only in this way the other doctors would learn to be aware of the need for this new approach in health care. The patients must take responsibility and demand a different approach to their treatment.

In saying no, he would not only help himself, but also help the system to change.

He stood up relieved he is not responsible for everything and everyone. He was right to say no sometimes, and to work out a better life for himself. Confrontation and visibility are needed to cause change. This experience reflected what was my own issue along the same lines. No one is helped if I have a breakdown simply because I have not learned how to say 'NO'. I had to stay in my integrity. My inner Gorilla needed to be activated. Maybe I will cause an upheaval, but it could not be avoided. I had to dare to face the chaos if that is what it will take to change things.

I was again reminded of the same lesson in another dream (Chapter 16: Dream nr 32: I let go of everything) around the same time. I was again at a shopping mall where I was to have a cup of coffee in a large restaurant. I approached a big, dark and heavy wooden table with all the coffee pots. The restaurant was a solid, old distinguished place. I suddenly noticed the table with the coffee pots was about to collapse. I had to stand there and hold it up, but it was getting way too heavy, so I asked one of the staffs to help me. He did not want to – or did not care. I suddenly got so mad that I simply let go and everything fell on the floor with a bang. I left the venue, surprisingly without feeling any guilt. I only felt relief and victory that I finally let go. This table was not my responsibility.

This dream made it clear how ready I was to let go of responsibility that did not belong to me. A big shopping mall with a restaurant is a collective place, a communal area. The restaurant seemed older and reputable, this to me represents old, conservative ways and attitudes. The staff member only reflected to me what I really wanted to do; to let go. Would it be accepted? Maybe not, but I knew I had to take the consequences of my choices.

I think the reward for conformity is that everyone likes you, except yourself.
– Rita Mae Brown

My body undeniably needed sunshine and warmth, so I chose to take a trip to Madeira that is a beautiful island out in the Atlantic Ocean. A cheap and easy solution I thought. The first day of this vacation I sat at an outdoor café overlooking the vast ocean. It was a beautiful place on the coast with flowers and palm trees all around. The sun reflected in the water and sent golden rays towards me. I enjoyed every second of the beauty and the feeling of freedom. I had such a great time that for a moment there I wondered if it truly was happening. A thought struck me that maybe I should 'be somewhere else' – or 'do something else'? Did I have something 'to do' that I was not seeing? This self-sabotage was so typical. These thoughts unsettled me so I said a silent prayer and asked for a clear answer if I was supposed to be somewhere else – or if I should simply stay and enjoy the time. Then I looked out over the ocean again enjoying the horizon and the blue sky without a cloud. Right above me I spotted a bird laying quietly on the airflow. It was not moving. I have seen birds floating on an airflow before, but usually you see small movements. This bird did not move at all and stayed there at the same spot. Slowly it dawned on me that this was the answer, 'Simply sit there and enjoy the view! Let go of everything else. Enjoy this beautiful place and moment in time! Simply receive it!'

The ego lives off time, Eckhart Tolle writes. The ego cannot feed off the moment. We will never be able to experience the feeling of freedom at any moment within the parameters that the ego, our conditioned self, demands. Once again, I had to acknowledge that *the time is working for me and not against me.* I really do not have to force myself to do anything. I must learn to stay anchored in the now, and simply flow, it is a matter of trust.

As I returned to my hotel room in the evening, I turned on my cd player and laid down on the bed for a moment of meditation. There was no music. I heaved a sigh and sent a prayer to the universe to help make the player work, as I really wanted some music while meditating. I checked the batteries and realised that they were dead and removed them. A little disappointed I laid back down again to meditate without music. As I closed my eyes and breathed calmly, I suddenly heard music coming from the player. There were no batteries in the player, but that did not seem to matter to the universe. I smiled and said thank you! Magic is not rational.

The laws of the universe of cause and effect show every response will hold the energy of the cause alive. If I do not dare to believe in miracles, they will not happen. If I let fear rule, I create pain, and if I defend my reaction the chain reaction will never end. I have the power to stop anything and create everything.

Chaos is created when I do not want to recognise who I am deep inside. For a moment I wonder what the larva must think when it is inside the cocoon going through the transformation. Does it think it soon will be a butterfly, or does it wonder if it will become a beetle? It would be chaos in the universe if the larva resisted and wondered what the outcome of the process would be like we do. It simply exists.

I am standing next to a tree with my palms touching the trunk of the tree, listening and wondering if the tree has anything to tell me. "Ask me why I am a tree" was the response. So, I did, and the tree answered, "Because I am a tree." It was that simple. I had to smile. Trees obviously do not have egos creating chaos with fearful questions. They know who they are and become who they are. I am light. *Light* heals and raises awareness. In this lies great power. I am a Dreamer and I was given more insight in my dormant Power.

I had a dream (Chapter 16: Dream nr 33: Fighting a monster) where I had travelled far and had finally arrived – I was finally 'home'. It was late in the evening and I was in California. I walked into my house and closed the door when I suddenly discovered there was a monstrous man standing behind the door. He was an executioner, a huge and fearsome troll. He was holding up a big old-fashioned axe over his head, ready to fell. He took a step forward to block the doorway so there was no way to escape. His intention was obvious. He was about to kill me. I realised I had no other choice than to summon the power from within. I lifted my hands and sent a powerful ray of light towards him. The power in the beam was so strong I had to use all the strength I could muster to keep my hands up while the light flowed towards the man. Suddenly the monster shrank into a small, scared boy. I was exhausted and asked him to leave. But he said that he was afraid to walk home alone. I let him convince me and followed him part of the way. "But now you have to manage on your own the rest of the way," I told him. Then I woke up with a feeling that I had overcome something enormous. A big adversary within had been defeated.

The monster was the essence and core of all my old fear-patterns and expectations that had manifested throughout a long life or many lives. In my dream I confronted and exposed the eternal and bothersome problems that I could not run away from. Now I could see the monster as the common denominator in all the times I had allowed myself to feel I had been abused, exploited, betrayed and rejected. It was now all exposed and defused. These thoughts no longer had power over my life. I was no longer a victim and reclaimed my power and space. The light in me revealed the monster to be a small, scared boy. He was the sum of all my illusions. Enough is enough. I accept my own authority and healing power.

I could see the connection between different events, places and teachings in my life now. I was carried forward on eagle wings. From this perspective, it was easier to see the overview. Things started to make sense to me.

Africa got me in touch with my feelings as well as my intuition and creativity. The childhood in Africa nourished me with play, mystery and hidden powers. I absorbed nourishment from nature and sensed everything around me without really being conscious of what I was doing. I experienced deep sorrow and incredible joy. In Africa we always admired everyone else in the great big white world. I remember the Africans reaction when we told them about white men landing on the moon. "There's nothing strange about that. The whites know everything, so why can't they land on the moon?" they replied, without the anticipated wonderment or enthusiasm.

Norway raised my awareness through adversities. I learned to use my analytical and mental powers. I had been lacking the words to express everything I knew deep inside. I received strength and the tools to confront myself and my life. The resistance I experienced here made me aware, mature and strong. In Norway, they say, "You shouldn't think that you are somebody special." You are not supposed to think you or others are special in any way. We are not good at celebrating our greatness. The critic is always lying in wait to give you an overhaul and lives comfortably in Norway. Here is where I learned to know and reveal my strong inner critic.

America was in the coming years going to teach me to follow *the Dreamer* in me. Here I was to be inspired to follow my heart and believe in my dreams. Here I was also going to learn the art of manifesting what I wanted. With self-love and love towards Mother Earth I would dare to communicate who I truly am. I was to learn how to see and embrace the colours and beauty in me. In the States it is important that you 'believe that you are somebody'. If I put forth an idea, I am met with encouragement and help, but only if I believe in myself and my success. If you fail, they drop you like a hot potato, I am told. 'You must believe in yourself. You must believe in your dream,' was the mantra I got from there. This gave me buoyancy to my wings.

How wonderful my life tapestry was working out. The gifts continued to flow towards me. The only thing that was holding me down and making it hard to receive all the gifts was old guilt…

Chapter 17
Forgive

An eye for an eye will make all blind.

– Gandhi

If I were to take the leap to my freedom, I had to forgive and let go of everything that had hurt me or I have exposed myself to. I realised this was the last step I needed to take, but it was as if I was waiting for permission from myself.

My body still showed there was a few more things to let go of. The body does not lie. My left knee was hurting, and I asked the healer Katherine Gyldenrose for help. She guided me into a deep meditative state through focusing on my breath. As I entered a quiet calm, I was asked to go into the pain in my knee. Suddenly I found myself standing on top of a wall overlooking a Mediterranean town with white houses. I was a female warrior leading my people, but I was deeply worried. A dark force was about to invade the town. Suddenly I started to cry. I realised I would fail the people I was set to lead. I could not stand up against the strong, dark resistance and watched a wave of dark-clad warriors on black horses take over my town. Then everything turned black.

As I returned from the meditation, I realised I had to let go of a deep-rooted pattern of shame and guilt about failing others and myself. The pain in my left knee stands for stubbornness and inflexibility. Pain is always telling us about resistance, and the left side can mean experiences of the past and of the feminine aspect of me. The memories of shame and fear were stored in my cells.

In my stubbornness I had *forgotten to pray for help when I needed it*. I had to learn to *work with* the Universe and Spirit in everything. Only then would I be able to stand in the battle and set myself free, to save and forgive myself! To be able to 'Receive' my power, my Sun and my inner Gorilla, I had to 'Release' my fear of failure. I had an 'aha' moment when I realised throughout my whole life I had tried to compensate for this seeming betrayal, and therefore I have taken on the responsibility for others. I thought I had to protect them and in doing so betrayed myself. At this time, I received several dreams and experiences guiding me through the process of forgiving.

Nobody can break your heart if you love yourself.

– Don Miguel Ruiz

The more responsibility I take for what is happening to me, the easier it becomes to forgive. At this point I had a dream (Chapter 17: Dream nr 34: Four emeralds lost) where I am travelling by ferry. I had bought four big and beautiful emeralds that were tear-shaped green jewels. Two were hanging with the pointed end down, the other two were pointing up. It seemed a man had taken my credit card and misused it on this trip. Because of this misuse the owner of the ferry reclaimed the jewels. I was desperate and exasperated that the company had allowed this man to use my credit card without checking his credentials. I was offered four new stones but said 'no thanks'. They were not as beautiful or valuable as mine. While I was mourning my loss, the original jewels suddenly appeared. This made me so relieved and happy that I started to cry. I woke up sobbing.

The ferry symbolises an emotional journey or process on the collective level. Four gems had been taken from me. My name Gro has four as its numerology 'destiny-number'. The number four stands for grounding, beauty, harmony, balance and creativity. The fourth energy centre in my body is the heart. If my heart fills with these qualities, it will always be protected. I had not protected my gifts and therefore made it possible for a mental male-energy to misuse the credit card, which (in Europe) is like my identity card.

The gems were potentially in balance as in my hidden gift, my treasure chest that is protected by the planet of Saturn. (Saturn in the sign of Libra that stands for harmony and balance). When I understood what I had lost, and the reason why they were taken from me, the valuable gems finally were returned. I received a second chance to take care of who I really am.

Nothing can be taken from me without my permission – conscious or unconsciously. This was a painful recognition. If I do not take care of what is me and mine, I am taking part in creating 'predators'. To forgive myself is the most difficult thing and knowing I had created it all was devastating.

Forgiveness is a mystical art, not a reasonable one.

– Caroline Myss

I was part of a small meditation group. One evening, a person in the group took it upon herself to confront me with something she felt was bothersome regarding my conduct. Usually I am a peaceful person but this time I got upset. I do not like to be criticised. Who does? Despite this, I do appreciate listening and learning about myself. A shadow side of mine is to be impatient, and I believe this is what she triggered. Several times she had domineered the group, commanding our time and attention. At one point I lost patience and my reaction was disproportionate. That night I had a dream (Chapter 17: Dream nr 35: Healing my heart) where a beautiful and strong woman was standing beside me. She had a warm and colourful personality and pointed two fingers at a certain spot on my back, right between the shoulder blades. She was standing there expecting and waiting for me to receive the healing she was directing at back of my heart. I felt a bit pushed, but she gave the impression she had all the time in the world. She was willing to wait for me, no matter how long it would take. When I understood this, I felt a great relief and trust. Then the tears came from deep within and I let go of all resistance. I woke up, wet with tears running down my face, thankful and calm.

I knew one of my strongest negative patterns was impatience, towards both myself and others. I realised it alone created a lot of pain. If I only were able to accept everything in the moment and be in the present, the pain in my life would less. In this dream two fingers stands for the duality. The spot on my back where she was holding her fingers was right over the back of the heart centre. The back symbolises the past. Now, I must forgive myself for all self-criticism throughout my whole life. I know it has been difficult for me to accept it has taken so long to heal. I realise I have awakened from several of these dreams crying. It is a good thing; a deep cleansing of the heart is happening.

Healing comes from gathering wisdom from past actions and letting go of pain that the education cost you.

– Caroline Myss

We only project what we have inside, and we own all our reactions. Now, as I had gone deep within and found both the light and the darkness within me, I found I was not so afraid anymore of being revealed. Then I got tested – again.

"Are you a walk-in?" I had been invited to a conversation group, where a man asked me this strange question.

I answered "maybe", with a smile – wondering whatever it meant.

"You are an angel and you have four large angels with you," said a woman as she passed me in a big hall. I simply received what she had to say and said thanks and Amen.

"You are cynical," a lady in a completely different setting told me.

"Okay," I replied and accepted that this was what she saw. I was not to take anything of it personal, I thought.

One day I received a long E-mail from a friend. Suddenly she was fed up thinking that I had not given her the attention she deserved. She wrote a whole page with terribly negative descriptions of who she thought I was. She could not find one good thing to say about me. We had many good times together for quite a while, but it did not seem to make a difference at this stage. She described me as a monster. Strangely enough, I noticed I did not have any big emotional reaction when reading the letter – except for wondering if I had really read this right?

I replied in short and friendly terms that I was very thankful for the nice times and experiences we had enjoyed together and then let go. A deep peace and thankfulness filled my heart that I had been led calmly through this test, as it could have hurt me deeply. I had not entertained her drama. Maybe she had been through a dark night with herself while writing the Email, I thought.

The stronger I grow, the stronger the tests become. My dreams dug deeper. They gave me more but also required more. When old 'pain bodies' appeared, I could handle them with less fear. I had accepted they are of my creation after all, and I was ready to forgive myself.

One night I had a dream (Chapter 17: Dream nr 36: Woman asking for help) where I was visited by a dark-haired woman. She was asking for guidance and help. She had been sent to me by the man she was now living with. It turned out to be the man I had been married to and now was divorced from. He had remarried but, in this dream, he seemed to have a mistress (again). That did not surprise me, I thought. I did not really relish the task, but still took on the challenge, as I knew I could handle it. I took notice the woman did not realise what she was doing to herself, and the relationship she was in was the reason for her problems. I gave her a clear and gentle description of the pattern she was struggling with. Then I told her with a loud and clear voice, "You do not want to accept this anymore!" I woke up and as I know every person in my dream is mirroring an aspect of me, I realised I no longer allowed myself to be in the role of victim. I will not let myself down again. I forgave myself, am true to and appreciate myself. I understood the dream possibly also was telling me about my relationship to other women. I most likely had been carrying suspicious and hurt feelings about not trusting women. They had seduced my husband or allowed themselves to be seduced. I forgave and accepted my responsibility.

Mentally, I had realised a lot at this time, but my body told me the emotions were still deeply wounded. The fibromyalgia gave me a daily reminder life was not as I wanted it to be. The strong outbreak of psoriasis in my hands and under the feet did not let go either. I was ready for *the deepest wounds to heal* and let go of what caused them.

As if ordered I had another dream (Chapter 17: Dream nr 37: Deadly wounded), and it shook me to the core. It was one of the most painful things I have ever experienced dreaming; I was lying on a square stone block, deep down in a catacomb-like room. I was lying on my tummy because my back was a mess through torture. It was like a great open wound. I lie there helplessly. Above me was a huge glowing hemisphere, about six or seven feet in diameter. It was made of rose-crystals and emanated a pulsating light shining over my whole body. I realised I was receiving healing from this dome. I was standing at a distance and watching myself in shock and fear, surprised that I was even alive.

With deep compassion and forgiveness, I was thinking, *Dad doesn't understand the great pain life has given me. He cannot understand.* I looked at the healing glow from the lamp and was surprised at the lack of 'feelings' in this source. It was neutral and healed unconditionally.

As I woke up, I sensed a deep tenderness towards myself. I knew I had to take good care of this dream. After a deep meditation, I allowed myself to open to the message of the dream. The back carries us and keeps us upright. The life force flows through the spine, and all experiences and emotional memories settle in the back nerves and muscles, tendons and neural pathways. It is like a memory board containing all we have experienced, and therefore also represents the past. On this stone table my emotional body was lying total smashed.

The thought that 'Dad' had not understood what I had been through made me sad. The mental male mentality in society (and in me), lacking in empathy and understanding had almost killed me. I had allowed a mental insensibility to become the authority and tyrant deciding my choices.

Now, I was so destroyed I had no other choice but to lie there and receive help.

Rose quartz symbolises divinity, feminine and unconditional love. The quartz lamp shines over my broken back (my life) and heals it. 'The power' in the lamp does not ask if I deserve help. There is nothing to forgive, I understand. It does not condemn. It heals unconditionally! I understand the Universe has no objections to my wishes. Like the genie in Aladdin's lamp the power says, "Your wish is my command!" It does not judge. What I believe it creates. The Universe is not personal - but reactive. It simply just gives me what I think and believe.

I forgave myself for having believed all the negative thoughts about myself and asked for strength to release them. I was ready to break free. I wanted to live!

The Butterfly:

I was breaking out of my self-created boundaries to try my newfound wings. I am lifted high upon the Sky to see my purpose on the Blue Rainbow Bridge, the road of wisdom. It is time to receive my beauty-self, and share the Power of my sun.

The light brings the colours of my Wings to be shared with the world.

The butterfly testifies of God's wonders, beauty, joy, love and the everlasting cycle of transformation.

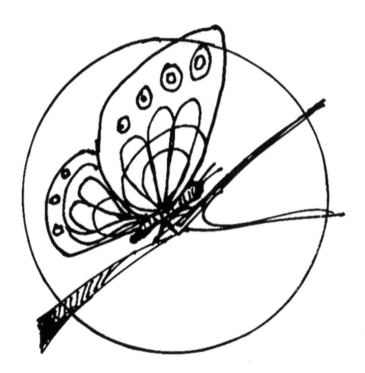

Chapter 18
The Flow of Life

Ego says, "Once everything falls into place, I'll feel peace." Spirit says, "Find your peace, and then everything will fall into place."

– Marianne Williamson

'Let go and let God' so clearly explains the fundamental criteria to allow a free flow of Life Force. Let go of the resistance and allow Life to support you.

Things inside of me were really starting to fall into place and one night I dreamt (Chapter 18: Dream nr 38: Granted a loan of 3 mill) I had been granted a loan of 3 mill. Norwegian kroners. I was standing in front of a cash register where I was to be given the money. The woman at the register asked if it really was true that I had been granted such a large amount and if I could document it? I became indignant. Of course, I had the documentation needed, I said and showed her a letter of reference. Then I woke up.

You are your own worst enemy, they say. I had been working hard and long to get through the resistance of believing I deserved to get well, have a stable economy and good and loving relations. In the dream one aspect of my personality still reflects I am not altogether sure if I deserve it. The number 3 shows the creative principal and unconditional service of love. Its energy is seated in solar plexus, the centre for self-esteem and strength. I need to believe; I deserve it all – unconditionally. All the zeros behind the number 3 express the energy of divine, creative and intuitive female power. In the dream it seems to me like the gift is a loan. I will have to account for my gifts and talents eventually. I forgave my internal critic and allowed myself to believe I can do what I put my mind to – and deserve everything I receive.

The day after having this dream, I happened to see a cute and thought-provoking movie, *The Magic Toy Store*. Mr Magorium, played by Dustin

Hoffman, owned a magical toy store where all the toys were alive. A young girl named Molly works in the shop and loving it. Henry, who is a young meticulous accountant, has a hard time believing in the magic of the shop. The owner, Mr Magorium, knows his time is soon over, as he is turning 243 years old, and wants to give this magic shop to Molly. This left her in despair because she has not faith in her own inner magical power.

For a long time the shop had been the only safe point of reference to a little boy called Erik. He tried eagerly to convince Molly to take over the shop. But she answered, "I can't be a kid anymore". Little Erik sees that she has the gift and needs to use it and says, But that's why Mr Magorium gave it to you. At last Molly let go of the fear and allow her inner child to breath her fresh life into the shop and all the toys come to life again.

Miracles are natural. When they do not occur, something has gone wrong.
— Marianne Williamson

At last, one day I was finally granted disability benefits! The back payments from the years it had taken for the case to be finalised were added. I was open to receive now and then it all came through! At this time, I realised I had to have new surroundings and a change of air to get well. I had been invited to US by a friend who was to marry an American in New Jersey. As the airplane circled over New York before landing, I suddenly had the sensation I had come home! *Strange,* I thought. There was no explanation why I should feel like that. Something inside me was very touched by the return to this foreign city.

My friends were to get married the next day and I was the maid of honour. That evening I suddenly got terribly ill and went to bed early. I felt a major flu approaching and the fever knocked me out completely. *What poor timing*, I thought despairingly. Throughout the night the fever rose, and I was really having a hard time. Half asleep, I suddenly noticed a strong light coming through the window to the left of the bed. A blueish beam of light moved over my body. With a strange buzzing it moved towards the lower part of my tummy and stayed there for a long time. I was lying there quietly and puzzled, just allowed it to happen. I could feel the buzzing throughout my body where the light was working. It dawned on me I had been healed. Then I fell asleep and slept peacefully through the rest of the night.

As I woke in the morning I was completely healed, without a trace of illness or cold, not even a little sniffle. My friends commented with amazement how well I looked this morning.

They had not expected this, as they pointed out I really had not looked well the night before.

Without getting into the details, I jokingly said I had been visited by an UFO and that did the job. They would not have believed it anyway and I did not need their approval, I thought.

Something here in the States heals me. I was at the right place at the right time. The illness was a message there was something I needed to get cleansed within me before entering new and important relations the next day.

When I think about what the 'Power of Light' has done for me, I am reminded of an American clairvoyant who lectured in Oslo a couple of years earlier. He had been working for the American government and the CIA for many years. He had defected and was 'laying low', as he expressed it. I 'checked out' his energy and he seemed a bit frightening to me. I did not really understand why. Maybe it was because he was dressed all in black, I thought to put my mind at ease. He was standing in front of the crowd and scanned the audience as he nodded in my direction, smiled at me and said, "You don't have to be afraid." I got so embarrassed. Apparently, I am easy to read. The explanation of why I had felt the way I did came when he said he had to admit that for many years he had been working for 'dark forces'. He had allowed the intelligent services use 'his gifts' as a clairvoyant to spy on and expose both enemies and friends. He had been successful and was slowly pulled deeper into matters that he couldn't justify to himself. He finally pulled out, but this was not with the support or acceptance from his former employer. He explained at this point that he did not feel very safe. He still had a lot of sensitive information. Still, he travelled far and wide to tell about his experiences and about the power and gifts that he had abused. He felt responsible to talk about how we could protect ourselves against such manipulation. He said, "If we get centred and fill up and surround ourselves with light it's the only thing that can withstand the negative forces and thought manipulation. Think and feel you are filled up with light! Stay in this light. This is the only protection that works."

I returned to Norway after the trip to my friends in New Jersey. But Just a few months later I returned to the States again. I brought a friend Myron this time and left for LA, California. I knew I was there for a special reason but did not yet knew what it was. I just knew I would be led. One day, Myron found a lot of reading material when going out food shopping in a health food store. He fell ill and had to stay in bed and therefore got me something to occupy my time. Very thoughtful of him. I thumbed through a magazine called Body, Mind and Soul. And here I discovered close by in Pasadena this weekend there was a Body, Mind & Spirit Expo. Well, *maybe that is why I came here*, I thought. It really was the only thing I wanted to do right then.

I stepped into a great hall where the energy was calm, clear and with a good overview. I walked around and took in all the impressions. Then I decided to get a reading from Laura Lee. She is a young woman who looks like an angel and tells me she communicates with angels, and she channels.

I sat down, and she holds my hands in hers while quietly closing her eyes. It looks like she is praying. Then, only knowing my name, she says: "You will soon live here. You will not have to work for your income. I hear drumming. You will have success with your paintings here. You have wonderful gifts as a healer."

I sit there in shock, tears streams down my face. She does not know I come from Norway. She does not know I am an artis, and that I now receive disability benefits or had been working as a healer for years. She does not know anything about my upbringing in Africa, where I every evening fell asleep listening to the sound of drums from the village. She has no idea my greatest desire right now is to be able to live here in CA for some time.

I felt received as if they expected me here and felt deeply relieved by this confirmation. During my stroll throughout the hall I struck up a conversation with Diana Payne, an astrologer who reads Tarot cards. She spotted me at a distance and strangely enough I felt drawn to her.

"How wonderful to meet a sister," she said with a big smile while she pointed out the similarities between us. I saw we had a few of the same physical characteristics, maybe we did on an energetic level as well? We talked for a while and then she laid some cards for me. After she had done the reading I left, thinking she was incredibly good, as she described an earlier relationship I had and gave a very fitting description of what happened. I also received some constructive guidance regarding what she could see coming up ahead. I thanked her and let the things she said settle, way back in my subconscious. I better simply take one day at a time, I thought.

After a few weeks in Los Angeles, I returned to Norway and my friend Myron headed home to Minnesota. It took another year and a half before I was back in California. This time I was travelling on vacation with my friends from New Jersey, the couple that was married. They treated me to a week in Palm Springs and then we left together for Los Angeles. Again, totally unexpected, there was a Body Mind Spirit Expo close by.

As I entered the big hall, I again saw Diana Payne, the astrologer from last time. I saw she was busy and looked around while waiting for her. When she was free, I came around smiling and a bit embarrassed, I carefully approached her. She would not remember me I thought. But she jumped up and gave me a big hug. I was very touched and thankful. Strange and at the same time genuinely nice to be recognised and received so warmly – again.

Laura Lee, the angel reader that I had a session with last time, had a lecture this day that I wanted to attend. My friends wanted to join me. Laura Lee was going to tell about her work and communications with angels. The lecture was to be about half an hour and then she would open for channelling for the audience. My friends and I sat towards the back of the huge hall. As Laura Lee starts channelling, a soul is stepping forward who shows up to be the sister of an elderly, very tired woman in the hall. She receives correct information, confirmation, guidance and comfort from her deceased sister. The lady who received this help, sat down, very moved.

Now, only fifteen minutes were left of the allotted time Laura Lee had. She asked for someone in the hall who knows a diseased artist called Johan. She seems a little insecure as it is a name, she has a bit of a hard time with. Quietly I have asked higher powers for a message, confirming if I was on the right track in my life. No one is responding, and Laura Lee is still struggling with the name, but then she mentions Carl, and it still has to do with fine art, she says. I get slightly panicked. My teacher at the art school in Trondheim, 25 years ago, was called Carl Johan. He died the year after I moved from the city. Could it be him? I slowly raise my hand afraid this could be a total miss. Laura motioned me to come up. She acknowledges my reluctance but reassures me that if I just come up, we'll figure out if this is the right contact. I walked up on stage a little uneasy. She right away confirms that I am the person this soul wants to contact. Then she looks surprised at me and exclaims "Is it you? Are you really back?" She wraps her arms around me while I was shaken and deeply moved to receive this heartfelt reception. This truly is strange. Laura Lee meets thousands of people every year through her workshops and performances all throughout the States. She had met me for about ten minutes one and a half years earlier. How in the world could she remember me? As I stand there on stage, stunned, she says this departed soul is immensely proud of what I am doing.

"He says you are doing something completely different now?" That was correct, as I had been his student learning sculpting. Now, I had been painting and teaching intuitive painting for years. "He really supports you in your choices," she said. "He is one of your guides. He is excited about the fact that you have the courage to do what you want now – and set yourself free from other's expectations." Carl Johan Flaate was, as mentioned earlier, my teacher in sculpting at the art school in Trondheim. The fact that he came through was incredible touching. He had meant so much to me. Life was full of synchronicity and magical flow and showed me I was not alone.

After one week in Los Angeles, my friends returned to New York, and I had to find a reasonable place to live by myself. I was dropped off at a crossing in the middle of LA by a Starbucks. I walked in and asked if I could leave my luggage there while trying to find lodging. That was no problem. How nice and friendly, I thought.

To find a suitable hotel was more difficult than I had expected. I am an optimist but not always a realist, some would say. After having looked for a while without finding anything, I decided to go to a five-star hotel. They realised I was not out to find a hotel in their price range and offered to find a taxi driver who could help me. This was exactly what I had hoped for. They told me this taxi driver knew the area well. He was a nice, elderly grey-haired Indian. He was friendly and would help, they reassured me. We picked up my luggage at Starbucks and set out on our search. Stopping by many hotels, I would jump out to check the prices while he waited in the car. But none of them were within my price range. After a long while, the driver turned up a driveway to a place I was sure I could not afford. The old Indian told me to still go in and try. The line was long at the reception, and I was worried about the taximeter. I looked around in the lobby and was sure I could not afford this and walked out. The driver was standing by the taxi, talking with one of the uniformed porters. I sat down in the car. "Well, how did it go?" the driver asked me.

"That was a waste of time." I replied. The taxi driver had informed the porter about my situation while waiting for me.

"Wait a minute!" the porter said and went into the reception. Shortly after he returned with the hotel director that greeted me with a friendly smile and asked what I was looking for. I told him the price range I could afford and added I would need a room for 14 days. It turned out the price I mentioned was half of what they normally ask. The director thought for a while and then accepted my request. If I would stay the 14 days, we had a deal! I lived like a king with all the service afforded a fully paying guest for fourteen days. What a miracle! The old Indian gave me his card – in case I would need further help in the future. I had a lifeline and felt safe once again.

I meet angels everywhere. They say, if you acknowledge the help that you receive, you will get more! I am not alone on this journey! I rest in the flow of life and allow it to take me to a perfect place, for the perfect price and at the perfect time. I then return to Norway to prepare for the longer trip to the States. I had decided to 'go with the flow' toward my big dream.

Chapter 19
America – and the Big Dream

And those who were seen dancing were thought to be insane by those who could not hear the music.

– Angela Monet

After having sold my apartment and given away everything I owned, I said goodbye to friends and family. I was 58 years old and boarded the plane to the States. With two suitcases and some 'airy plans' I set out on my long-awaited journey. I was going to Bandon first, this little magical place, south in Oregon by the West Coast. This was the place I had found in such an extraordinary way on my earlier travel in the States.

Bandon received me with open arms. On the first day, I found the small bakery in town. Here I had a fresh and tasty pastry and a good cup of coffee. Suddenly a lady showed up by my table. She greeted me, very friendly, presented herself as the mayor of the town, and wondered if I was the Norwegian lady looking for a place to live? Someone from my hotel, as it was the only hotel in town, had told her about me. Surprised I affirmed that I was. The mayor had a small vacant house only a stone's throw away. She even to let me borrow one of her cars if I wanted. She had several. I could rent everything for only a few hundred dollars.

'Someone' must have prepared the way for me. It seemed a little odd, as if I was expected and everything was planned and ready to receive me. I was now being forced to let go of old expectations of rejection and loss that have resided so deeply in me through my whole life.

There are black ravens everywhere here. They jump out in front of me on the path and crisscross in the air above me. I almost feel trailed. It is fascinating but also a bit scary. I decide to find what these bluish black birds symbolise. They say lack of understanding creates fear, so I decided to investigate what they were all about. In many fairy tales, we read ravens are the companions of witches. I therefore was pleasantly surprised when learning about the important spiritual role they play in different cultures. In the book Medicine Cards by Jamie Sams and David Carson I learn ravens are 'The Guardians of the Holy Laws'. They are considered messengers between the different consciousness levels and bring warnings regarding important changes. They often show up when we need to be reminded about "the laws of the Universe" and the fact that "we attract what we think about"! They warn us to be aware about our thoughts, in the moment. Bird represent what is happening on the thought level. I am receiving help to let go of all negative thought-patterns about myself, about these black birds, my life and my future.

I walked along the coastline and admired the forces of nature here. The wind grabs me and my thoughts. It forced its way into my head. "You have to let go even if you don't want to!" I seemed to hear! I was starting to understand what Bandon was supposed to help me with. My thoughts are to be blown clean! I was forced to let go of old junk, everything I no longer needed or enjoyed. Three words fell into place again: *Relax, Release, and Receive*!

I do not find it hard to get to know people in the States and enjoy the new acquaintances and quickly gain many new friends. One dear new friend is Suzanne who is a healer and massage therapist. She gave me a massage that forced consciousness into my body. I experienced her as an incarnation of Mother Earth, with her great, strong smile and her complete disregard for nonsense or the victim-mentality. She reminds me of what I know – but still work to integrating.

My story becomes insignificant compared to her pain story. She finds strength and pride in the fact that she survived. Almost completely freed from identifying herself with the pain story, she simply laughs about her own tragedy. I also want to come to this place within me. To laugh in the face of tragedy, just as the African women did. I want to find my African Sun within me. Suzanne's story is brutal. We both understand what it is all about and our friendship becomes important to me.

Suzanne lives in a small self-made house deep in the woods. It is not much to look at, but she is proud of it because she has put it together herself and turned it into a cosy little home. Here in this little spot in the woods she lives with some different animals that she has rescued and is caring for. Amongst the animals is a happy and frisky little dog with three legs who now has found a safe home. She has three horses. They are a bit nervous; she explains with a smile. She takes care of them and they are safe with her. Nature is rewarding her for taking care of it. So much love! I was slowly awakening to the importance of the love between nature and myself.

I received inspiration, support and guidance here in Bandon. Books from the local bookstore 'fell out' of the shelves and straight into my hands. They end up being the perfect recharging I needed. I received clear confirmations that I was at the right place at the right time. My spirit and body happily absorb new information and inspirations. I am reminded I am as safe as I allow myself to be.

One day on my way to the library it started raining heavily. The library was quite a walk from where I lived, and it was really pouring down. I sought cover as best as I could under my umbrella. A car approaches from the opposite direction. It was driving fast, and the water was spraying to the sides. But as it passes me it slows down and almost stop. An elderly woman rolled down the window and shouted something to me. It was hard to hear what she was saying because of the rain, so I stopped. She shouted that she was simply wondering who I am, and where I am from? I had to laugh and shouted back that I come from Norway! She let go of the steering wheel and clapped her hands, laughed out loud and wished me welcome! Then she closed the window, waved and drove off. I am noticed, I thought, and chuckled!

I so enjoyed meeting real, happy and unvarnished passion! Finally, I had found a place where people could laugh out loud and show childlike joy and enthusiasm. I felt the African side of me was waking up. It was welcomed here. Strangely enough this small place has a quite sizable art gallery with a whole section devoted to art from West Africa. To me this was a rare and strange coincidence which gave me the impression that I had come around 'full circle'. I bought a beautiful 'sun mask' from Cameroon, reminding me of my African sun: a memory of two worlds meeting. Downtown Bandon has only two short streets, but still offer all you can wish for of pastries, food, art, handicrafts and the necessary assortments of clothing. It is a tiny place in the country, but I lack nothing here. People approach me with open hearts and a generosity I hardly ever have experienced before. Or is it I who finally am learning to receive?

Communication is to me an outstanding characteristic of the States and I have an opportunity to practice. They talk here. They talk to you whether you are a friend or a stranger. They greet your cheerfully and talk about the weather, the latest TV show and about a new product on the market. I enjoy it all. They are not frightened off by my smile and I find it easier to breath here. I am no longer on guard against criticism. My body is truly starting to relax.

Although there are only a few thousand people in Bandon, they have a theatre worthy of a larger town. It appears to be a well-equipped and professional theatre with talented local actors. One weekend they put on a well-known classical American comedy. I had decided to experience and enjoy as much of the culture as I could manage, and I really enjoyed it all.

While waiting for the second act I had a glass of wine, when a lovely elderly couple approached me. "We just want to tell you that you are a very beautiful woman. Have you considered modelling?" At first, I wondered if it was truly me the elderly man was talking to, and then I had to strain not to burst out laughing about the unexpected compliment. The friendly sincerity in their faces forced me to pull myself together. I smilingly thanked them and said the thought had never occurred to me, as I was thinking of the fact I was soon turning sixty. They wished me a continued nice evening as they left me stunned and amused.

Well, honestly, I was touched to tears. Consider my situation, I was quickly approaching 60 and the last time I remember receiving a compliment regarding my looks was in Africa when I was around twelve or thirteen. I was home during vacation and was standing outside our house in the village called Mbe in the Duru valley where my parents were stationed at the time. An African college boy was standing there, waiting for something when he ventured out to compliment me. "A yeno yangpa sukre" he said with a grin.

"You are like white sugar." I impulsively hurled a rock at him. (I hope not too big.)

"Don't come here with such nonsense." I was irate. I did not feel pretty at all. I was quite sure it was an insult.

Did I have to go all the way to the West Coast of the United States, almost sixty years later, to hear that I was just a little bit pretty? That time in Africa did not really count, I thought. We were four sisters, and among my siblings I was counted to be the least attractive. That was the established fact with no objection from me. I believed this totally, even though it could have been my own thoughts. Perhaps it was enough that no one denied it. My self-worth was talking. Now it was time to change this self-talk.

In Bandon, I was identified by the residents as 'the Norwegian lady with the backpack'. Everything about me seemed special and intriguing. I felt seen and deeply appreciated. I could not avoid receiving the healing by the Joy of Life.

On the web page of a renowned doctor and healer from Oregon I read they have discovered a new energy centre or chakra. It is situated between the throat and heart. They call it the 'Clown chakra'. If you do not have an open mind to see the humorous in things, this chakra is closed. If one energy centre is closed it affects all the other energy centres throughout the body – it is like a chain reaction. This centre is just as important as all the rest!

The sense of humour is holy, I am learning now. I have started to use the empty garage where I am living as an atelier and paint a chubby turquoise elephant with small pink and transparent wings. It had been quite a few years since I painted, but now I was loosening up. I painted, played and laugh. My inner child experienced space and freedom of expression. Old thoughts and painful memories were blown away. The Sun within me awakened.

An old eccentric popped by and entertained me. He gave me a beautifully decorated piece of paper with his signature. It is a Reiki Healer certificate. He must have considered me worthy to be honoured with this gesture. Later, he arrived with two more certificates, this time for level two and three. I could see they were originals and understood he, sometime during his younger years, had been a Reiki Master. I soon was a certified Reiki Master myself – just like that. I just had to laugh. It was so ridiculous and fun at the same time. Maybe the Universe just wanted to give me some recognition.

While living in Bandon I was invited to go to Hawaii with my friends from New Jersey. Several nice things are simply falling into my lap at this point. Seems like I am ready to receive! Before I left Norway for Bandon, I had received a reading by a Norwegian expert on the Maya calendar. This is the Indian answer to our Western astrology. She explained my two main symbols are the 'Hand' and the 'Monkey'. The 'Hand' symbolises the creator and healer, and the 'Monkey' among other things, symbolises learning through play, movement and creativity. This was knowledge correlating with my own knowledge of myself. I asked her if she knew what symbol ruled the States and Hawaii? She accepted the challenge and entered further into her studies and discovered Hawaii is the "Hand" and the States is the 'Monkey'. Life plays around and laughs with me through synchronistic experiences. I had been taught synchronistic signs and happenings were confirmations. I gained strength and support from this endorsement. I concluded all was well.

The time in Hawaii, with its heavenly beaches, blue ocean and sunshine, nourished me and reached deep down into my soul with an injection of pure vitality and energy. It was as if the universe opened all the gates for blessings to pour towards me.

In the last couple of days I was in Hawaii, there 'surprisingly' happened to be a Body, Mind and Spirit Expo. This was as if ordered. As I toured the stands observing what was happening, I spotted a man who obviously was a native. He sat there completely relaxed and bare-chested in the heat. I could not see anything on his table, so I approached him and asked what he was doing here at the fair. "Do you want to hear?" he asked and stood up with a quiet, innocent confidence. I nodded and smiled. He closed his eyes, breathed deeply and then started a beautiful, deep chant. His voice raised and filled the room. He chanted for me and owned the space as he gave of himself to the point that it seemed the whole room was vibrating with a warm and healing power. This man was simply himself, anchored in his own power. Tears were running down my cheeks. When he finished and saw my tearstained face, he laughed warmly and said that it has this effect on people. I recognized it, I said, and smiled back at him through my tears. The natives of Hawaii are known for their relaxed unceremonious ways. Hawaii is called The Islands of Light. Light heals. He was a strong healer who had unconditionally given me of his power and gifts. I thanked him from my whole heart.

The night following this experience I dreamt (Chapter 19: Dream nr 39: A dream-visit) I was standing with a group of people in a small courtyard surrounded by some low buildings with an open gate towards the road passing by. It was a dark night, but the light from the lamps lit up the space where we were standing. I looked up at the starry sky and enjoyed the special atmosphere. My attention was suddenly drawn towards the gate. I noticed the shaman from the exhibition was passing by. He stopped and looked curiously at us and suddenly he was right there with us. He was dressed in a white and clean shirt, and I felt such warm joy and moved right next to him and gently put my head on his right shoulder, hoping quietly that he would not mind. I was filled with feelings of warmth, safety and calm as I breathed deeply and freely. I woke with a smile.

The next day was the last day of the fair as well as the last day of our stay in Hawaii. We returned to the exhibition as we wanted to join another lecture. I was walking around the hall while waiting for the lecture to start when the shaman from the day before noticed me at a distance and got up and waved eagerly to me. Without waiting for me to get to him, he shouted loud and uninhibited across the hall. "Did you dream about me last night?" I laughed, surprised and caught off guard by being exposed so publicly. He had no inhibitions. His open and liberating honesty touched me. I nodded back laughingly and giddy that I had. He waved, laughed warmly and nodded back with recognition. Neither of us needed to say more. I received it as I perceived it - a healing dream connection. We all are one and live in the same dream space. Now, I found it fun to live and the power within my Sun felt supported and grew stronger.

America helps me to believe I deserve to receive as everything is coming my way. Back in Bandon the town continues to protect and support me. To recognize I deserve joy and abundance is new. It is a concept that my inner being had resisted strongly for my whole life. An old superstition was changing now.

The universal laws challenge us to test them. We truly can create miracles. Miracles cannot be created through logic. They do not work through logic. I am painting and finding joy in the playful and creative process, while wondering why in the world I had allowed myself to be pushed through all the drudgery and striving. As an artist, I have learned if I do not have any expectations and simply set my inner child free, I often create the picture that is sold first at my art exhibition. The picture carries the energy I had when I playfully created it – a free and passionate flow of creativity has a tremendous magnetic power. Florence S. Shinn was an artist, art therapist and an author. She taught metaphysics several years in New York and wrote about interesting phenomenon of playfulness. The four most prominent artists in Philadelphia, the city where she's from, had one thing in common; none of them took their art solemnly. They had fun, played a lot and found great joy in simply creating. They were the four who eventually became the most successful with their art. "The riskiest thing you can do is not taking the chance" – I read on a cinema advertisement in passing. I reflected on this and understood: to take chance on myself was the challenge.

The movie 'Communication with God' is about Neale Donald Walsch's life. He was a significant spiritual leader, and he told the story that he had to get to rock bottom before being able and willing to receive help from Source. When he had nothing left to lose, he finally was empty enough for the 'voice' to break through. Then he became a tool for something far bigger than himself. He discovered his story had no other importance then the wisdom he gained from it. He knew the only thing he could do was to live in the now. His gift to the world is not his pain but his heart. It is a heart that is filled with 'God's voice' and he becomes a channel for this voice. This is only possible if he is present every moment.

Neale Donald communicates we only are and have what we believe that we are and have. "Give from your abundance," he said to a poor man. Then he reminds this poor man that his abundance possibly could be his heartbeat or his humour. Some years later Neale Donald meets this man again. He hardly recognises him because he is a well-groomed and rich man. "I did what you said – and look what it gave me," he said. He had just used his gift of humour, and that was the gift that gave back. 'Enthusiasm' means inspired by the gods, the true voice from the heart. Being one with God within. I had to dare to believe that I am enough and have the courage to live it. To live in integrity, like the Gorilla.

After six months in Bandon, my residence permits expired and I had to pack my bags and say goodbye to Bandon. One of my new friends had told me about a beautiful place in Mexico that she recommended. It was called San Miguel de Allende and was situated up in the mountains in central Mexico. My journey continued. Several magical and joy-filled experiences were awaiting me, and my heart was expanding.

Chapter 20
Joy Lifts

Sleep and dream of joy, and remember above all else, you feel good not because the world is right, but your world is right because you feel good.

– Wayne Dyer

It is evening and I am by the Pacific Ocean in Mexico, sitting on a beach beneath a dark sky covered with stars. While I relax in a beach chair, I munch on a small homemade pizza, and watch a movie projected on a white cloth gently wafted by the breeze. After two magical months in San Miguel Allende, deep in the highlands of Mexico, I was now in Sayulita, a small fishing village by the Pacific Ocean. Sayulita is a hidden spot with jungle all around except for this beautiful opening towards the ocean.

There I am. sitting alone under the dark starry sky, caressed by the warm ocean breeze. I am enjoying my freedom and the beautiful surroundings and the fact that I am the sole attendant at the cinema performance. I chuckle as I watch the "cinema manager" happily running the movie just for me, a movie that I was allowed to choose. The restaurant owner, also the cinema manager, has made the pizza according to my specific wishes. I giggle at the silly action movie I chose. I am practicing how to experience life playfully.

Walk as if you are kissing the Earth with your feet.

– Thich Nhat Hanh

When I visited, Sayulita was a hidden treasure in Mexico, years before the TV show 'Paradise' made it public domain. Many years ago, some European youth had settled here when they discovered it was a perfect spot for surfing. There were also many artists and spiritual awakened people who settled in the

157

aria. It mad for a rich culture. I had discovered a true pearl. The young couple who ran the hotel I was living at also had a gallery on the first floor. Here they sold pearl necklaces of their own design. They were also sold in New York and St Tropez. The pearls were gathered in the Pacific Ocean by divers they knew. I bought my first real pearl necklace as well as one for my daughter. Just because we deserved it!

Back, to when I arrived in San Miguel Allende, I landed at the airport about two hours by car from my destination. It was late at night, and I would be going into the mountains. Someone had cautioned me never to hire my own taxi in Mexico. This could be disastrous. I prayed a silent prayer that everything would work out okay. It turned out that the airport had their own taxis and they were supposed to be safe. I paid in advance and we headed out into the dark on a dusty road. They had no streetlights. The taxi driver explained our destination was a safe place, but we were to travel through a couple of villages where we could encounter problems. As we came close to the first village the taxi slowed down and we slowly and carefully passed a couple of trucks packed with soldiers armed to the teeth. We breathed a sigh of relief as we drove by without an incident and continued into the dark. I was speaking with the taxi driver in English although he did not understand much, while he in turn responded to what he believed I must have said in Spanish, which I did not understand. We communicated happily in this way for two hours.

Safely at our destination, I thanked him, relieved that all went well, and gave him a generous tip.

My accommodation was in a large holiday complex, but I did not care for it much. Next day, a lovely, balmy afternoon, I walked to central San Miguel. I sat down on a bench in a park and enjoyed the hustle and bustle around me. It seemed that both families and tourists congregated here and had a good time. Next to me were three American ladies around my age. We started talking and they told me they lived in a charming Bed and Breakfast called Art House only a few blocks away. "Why don't you move there?" they asked. Intuitively this seemed the right place for me. The owner of *Art House* was an American lady named Barbara from California. For two wonderful months, I enjoyed the company and fellowship of many lovely people who gave of themselves freely. I was warmly being taken care of and felt safe. I was invited to parties, the theatre and outings. We went to hot springs in the mountains where we relaxed in life giving spring water. I was nourished in body and soul and healing became quite apparent on my skin as well.

The evening when Obama was voted president in 2008, we were all gathered in the living room for election vigil and a party. This was so much fun! I found new friends here that will always be part of my life and this place on earth will always be a part of me.

San Miguel de Allende was founded by a Franciscan monk in 1542 It is built near a huge crystal vein but is also known for the silver mines close by. It is a small town but has an unusual number of churches and cathedrals and therefore on UNESCO's World Heritage list. I always visit churches on my travels – even if they are not of my faith. They have a story to tell and somehow help me connect to the place I am visiting. I find safety and peace there.

One Sunday I ended up in a Catholic Mass and watched the ceremonies and crowds of people with fascination. Everyone participated so actively and full of life, I thought, and discovered one of the reasons. The priest was leading the congregation in songs that Originated from many different religions.

Here everyone was obviously included. They were one.

With time I had learned to better sense, listen and be led. Barbara, the owner of Art House the Bed and Breakfast arranged for me to meet shaman Don Jesus in San Miguel. He was known beyond national borders. No harm in meeting him, I thought, and arranged one-hour appointment. As I entered the room, he asked me to sit down and he asked for my first name and date of birth. That was all he wanted to know. I sat there expecting a sign to indicate when he wanted me to talk or reply if he had any questions. But he sat there with his head in his hands and had seemingly no interest in me. There I sat in what seemed like eternity, but I felt relaxed. I knew he had to take the initiative. After a long silence I heard a few grunts and then he raised his head and snorted, "You are a large gorilla pretending to be a little girl!"

That was all he said. I really did not need to know anything else. I started to laugh. I was caught! My heart jumped in surprise and recognition. Instead of feeling hurt or offended I smiled and told him that he was right. This was strange. The message seemed so strangely familiar! We had a short back and forth conversation and then he said, "Come back when you have learned to say no!" That hit home also.

I returned to Art House Bed and Breakfast and sat deep in thought, thinking about the amazing coincidence between what I experienced with this shaman here in Mexico and the experience at the acupuncturist in Oslo a year prior, when I felt the huge gorilla taking place in my body. Don Jesus had seen it! *Now, I had to recognise it.* Of course, the same day I met someone who was to test me. She 'pushed' me to say 'yes' to do something I really did not have the energy to do. No surprise, I fell ill. I had to see the humour in it!

Once more I was reminded of my great lesson and what the Gorilla does so well: he holds his boundaries, lives in true integrity, playing and acknowledging who he really is. My spirit was lifted when I once more was reminded of my power and the creative Joy in my heart.

Chapter 21
Laguna

*The two most important days in your life are the day you are born and the day
you find out why!*

– Mark Twain

After three months in Mexico, I returned to Norway and celebrated Christmas
with my family, but after a couple of months I again returned to California. My
family lives in Norway, but I feel home in the States. I try not to get confused.
At this time, it was all about me and my journey! California was calling me and
so I returned.

For a couple of days, I lived in a small hotel by Venice Beach in Los Angeles.
I had stayed in the same area before and remembered the colourful and energetic
life unfolding at this beach.

I searched the net for a hotel by Laguna Beach that was one-hour drive south
of Los Angeles. I was advised *not* to go to Laguna Beach because it is so
expensive there. Last time I visited LA a couple of friends took me for a Sunday
ride to Laguna. It must be like a dream to live here, I thought at that time. Now,
I wanted to give this dream a chance and defy all objections. On top of the list I
found the first and cheapest alternative called Art Hotel. There was no need to
investigate any further. My curiosity was peaked, and I reserved a room. I did
not give it any further thought why I was so intrigued by this name. When I
arrived at the Art Hotel, I was again reminded there was something familiar about
the name but could not connect or remember what it was. They had named the
hotel about one month ago, the owner explained. "It's not much art to brag about
yet, but we'll get there," she added, a little embarrassed. Gail had a big heart and
liked to support local artists.

Gail was to become a dear friend. She helped me to find a nice flat, reasonable, and centrally located in Laguna. She kept an eye on me and helped me create a wonderful social network. Maybe that is why I was led to this place? I felt surrounded by angels and had found yet another paradise where I was received as a queen (Chapter 2: Dream nr 2: Meeting with elephants). I had arrived in the 'lagoon' from the dream (Chapter 8: Dream nr 9: Rainbow in the lagoon) long ago, where the rainbow reached out into the water and I had to defy the wind and rain to reach my treasure -out in this lagoon. That is what Laguna means – lagoon. I would find something valuable here. I knew it.

It dawned on me as I recognised the similarities between my host here in Laguna and where I stayed in San Miguel. Art House and Art Hotel had the same name almost and both had hosts that received me with open arms, as if I were a dear and expected guest. I was reminded of the time when I was studying fine art in Trondheim, and was provided free food and lodging by kind people. And then, also the generous offer from the mayor of Bandon in Oregon.

So much love and kindness in the world! If I act in trust, the universe responds with generosity!

Laguna Beach is surrounded by small hills protecting the surrounding world. Around the 1900, a group of artists settled in this idyllic place. As it grew, it got the reputation as 'The San Francisco of the South'. Today art and spiritual work coexist in a fruitful symbiosis. Laguna Beach is just as famous for its art galleries and art-exhibits as San Miguel de Allende is for its churches and cathedrals. Art and spirituality seem to go hand in hand in my life.

Laguna was teaching me about abundance, about joy in life and being easy going, while San Miguel taught me integrity, spirituality and community. I was nourished in body, mind and soul. Every place I was led to reflected joy and love.

One of the galleries in Laguna had a permanent exhibition of the works of author and illustrator Dr Seuss. The Cat with the Hat is one of his world-famous children's books. The gallery displays illustrations and paintings as well as his funny and imaginative sculptures of animals with humorous human features. Many of them wear weird hats. Dr Seuss had a big, secret hat collection which was discovered and put on display after his death.

I am reminded that we can choose to wear many weird, ridiculous and wonderful hats and imagine ourselves in many roles. Nothing needs to be serious.

My inner, playful child is nourished and given freedom to express herself now. I enjoyed my little paradise immensely, and by and by gained many new friends. Once more I was invited to enjoy much fun. I did miss my children, but they had promised to visit me throughout the summer. I was looking forward to that. I had a nice little place with space for them as well.

The months flew by. I hardly noticed. One day after a wonderful morning on the beach, I walked up the stairs leading to my kitchen. As I opened the door, a beautiful butterfly flew out from the kitchen and by me. It was completely black with golden yellow stripes by the edges. I wondered where it came from and looked around the apartment but could not find any explanation. Later, the same day, I was out enjoying the sunshine and again, I experienced a butterfly flying out of the kitchen as I returned home. I tried to find the source of where they came from, but with no results. The next day I experienced the same *two more times* – and it was the same type of butterfly. I had now counted four butterflies flying out of my apartment Life had shown me that if something happens repeatedly, then a strong message is associated with the experience.

The next night I dreamt (Chapter 21: Dream nr 40: A large butterfly) about a large, beautiful, turquoise butterfly. It covered both my palms and I held it gently and with great admiration. Then I opened the window in my bedroom, lifted it up and let it fly outside. As it opened its wings, the sun shone through two beautiful big eyes on the wings. Butterflies are best known as symbols of transformation, but they are also beautiful greetings from the other side.

Before I had this dream, I had been visited by those four butterflies flying out from my apartment.

In numerology, Four stands for grounding: balance, beauty, harmony and creativity. My name, Gro, is also connected to the number four. The colour black on the butterflies contains all colours and has great grounding powers plus the potential of creativity. The golden outline of their wings reminded me of the golden edging of the white cape that my daughter had given me in a previous dream (Chapter 12: Dream nr 17: I was in a basement). I interpreted this as a golden energy framing the power of gifts within. The four black butterflies flew out of my kitchen, a room that often symbolizes the heart. That is where the gifts are prepared for serving.

The fifth butterfly, which came to me in my dream was very large and had the colours of a healer. Turquoise symbolises healing and awareness. Five symbolises manifestation and wisdom, but also curiosity about life and freedom.

The butterfly, which came to me in a dream, was very large and had the colour and wisdom, but also freedom, change and curiosity about life. Like emerging from a cocoon, the butterfly flew out the window of my bedroom where it has been resting, protected in preparation for manifestation.

The window the butterfly from my dream flies out of symbolizes the eyes of my soul. The sun, the symbol of God's Spirit, is shining through the eyes on the wings. I am ready to see everything through the light of love and allow the spirit to enlighten my intuitive eyes. I was ready for something new, although not yet aware of what it would be.

These butterfly experiences were to play an important part in the following decisions I was about to make. I was lifted and guided to something completely new, but still so strangely well known.

I had given myself plenty of time to rest and enjoy the sun and beach, and now I was ready for new inspiration and knowledge. I went online to look for anything of interest happening but had decided it could not be further away than a couple of hours from Laguna. Then I happened to notice The Four Winds. This was a shaman school run by Alberto Villoldo, a medical anthropologist, Shaman and author. I had read a couple of his books several years back and had thought, if I were to learn more about shamanism it had to be his teaching I would like to study! My heart was pounding as I checked out where this school was located. For all I would know, it could have been on the other side of the States. Well, the school was two hours from Laguna and a new semester was just starting! I was magically supported and guided – again

"The Four Winds" holds some of their classes in a center located near the juncture of two southern California deserts. The aria is called Joshua Tree because the striking plants of the same name growing in the area. At this school, my power was confirmed, and I was given tools I have benefited from ever since. At this school, there is no escaping. We are all being confronted with the masks we hide behind. I got to practice what *true integrity* means. I learned to recognize in myself and others the roles we play as victim, helper and abuser. When I let go of those images, I am set free. Incomprehensibly free!

The course I attended is called 'Healing the Light Body' and is energy-healing taught by Incan shamans. The native Indian shamans in the Amazon and Andes call themselves Earth Keepers. They live in complete harmony with all living creatures and believe humankind simply is part of a large brotherly or sisterly relation to everything Mother Earth is about. Everything is alive, and everything is holy. They honour, respect and work together with the spirit in everything. The shamans can see, heal and can travel in time and between worlds. Where they can find knowledge and help. A shaman makes himself invisible by becoming one with everything. I wanted to learn this. I wanted to learn to live in harmonious unity with everything. I wanted to learn to love everything. I wanted to learn to love life.

We sat in a circle in the meeting room and took turns explaining why we were there. I intuitively answered: "To ground my spirit." This felt true to me. My relationship to Mother Earth had suffered and I wanted to heal this. I wanted to love the earth again and feel safe. I knew that is why I came.

One of the first exercises we had, was to learn to follow invisible tracks. Everyone received a rock which had been initiated by Peruvian shaman, Don Fransisco. He was there to help guide us. That morning, I woke up with a splitting headache which gradually developed to a crippling migraine. I do not experience this often and was surprised.

There we were sitting in a large circle as the teacher was telling us about what was to happen after the gathering. The stone we had been given was to be used to track and read each other. We were supposed give a reading to another person's by using the stone in tracking the person's physically, emotionally and spiritually body. This would be an exercise in working with our energy-body and would happen after this morning gathering. I knew this exercise would be taxing, but I also knew I could do it – if only I didn't have that crippling headache.

As our teacher continued talking, I closed my eyes, breathe deeply and let myself fall inward. There was nothing else I could do. As our teacher continued talking about the exercise, I closed my eyes, breathed deeply and let myself fall inward. I had to let go of the teacher and the rest of the group.

There was nothing else I could do at this moment. I had to allow my inner self to reveal to me why this was happening. As I held the stone in my hand, I said a little prayer to be shown what I needed to understand. Then my mind let go and I was in a peaceful place. Suddenly *I saw* a big eye painted on the stone I had in my hand. It was colourful and powerful. I could see I had big eyes like that in rows up along my body, on my forehead and in the palms of my hands. I was puzzled but then heard a clear voice saying, "Let the Spirit do it!"

I took a deep breath and opened my eyes, surprised, and knew that I would be guided. I was just to be a tool, a channel for the Spirit! Surprised I also discovered the headache was completely gone! This all happened within a minute as I simply let go of my ego. I had possible terrorized myself unconsciously by my own expectations, and this could have caused the terrible migraine. I only had to let all my senses be used by the Spirit. When we later got together to do the exercise, it went miraculously well and was clear and correct. In trust I allowed the Spirit to supply all the information needed – in a free flow.

I remember I recognized the eye on the tracking stone as the same strong and beautiful eye I had seen in my dream with the big turquois butterfly. The sun shining through the large, beautiful eye is Spirit – The "All Seeing Eye"! I am continually reminded to let the light shine through me, through every thought and action and to let it lead me at every moment. The reward for letting go of controlling is to experience life itself. I see this remind myself of what pattern of control that has caused illness and breakdowns. My stubbornness is deep rooted. I remind myself to breath and trustingly let go. To be free and strong I had to own it all as I am a part of all that is. As I am opening for acknowledging my weakness I also am opening to my potentials.

I heard a voice saying, "I am all that I don't want to be – but I am also all that I want to be!" To be free and strong I had to own it all as I am a part of all that is.

Back in Laguna I immediately faced the first exercise or test. I was at the bus depot in Laguna. Often I am the only white person there. leaning people of color take the bus here and we were patiently sitting on a bench in the sun. the bus was late. Right in front of me are two pigeons. They take hold of each other's beaks and start a tug of war. I have never experienced birds fighting like this and I watch the show with fascination. They are jumping around, pushing and pulling, and neither of them wants to let go. They seem to carry on forever. Bizarre, I thought. Then the bus arrived. It turns dangerously close to a corner where an Afro -American boy was sitting, leaning his backpack up against the wall. He screams out loud as the bus drove over his backpack. The boy had jumped up and was squeezed up against the wall. He was furious and as the bus stopped, he ran to address the bus driver who was a middle-aged woman. The boy shouted that she almost killed him. And then the ruckus started. The bus driver defended herself that the boy should never have been sitting there, while the boy wanted her to admit to hazardous driving. No one was able to board the bus as they were standing in the doorway and shouting accusations at each other, and none of them were about to let up. After a while I decided to approach the female driver and whispered to her that it would be wise simply to apologise, but she continued to

166

defend herself staunchly. Now, she would not even allow the boy on the bus. The boy was in shock and deeply hurt.

They were in a dreadlock. I asked to be allowed to board the bus while telling the boy and the others to wait outside. The driver closed the door behind me, and we had a talk. I could see her despair behind the anger and stubbornness. I told her that I understood she was scared, but she could not really punish the boy for what had happened. She had to apologise and admit her careless driving. I told her I would make sure the boy would not cause any trouble on the bus if she let him in. She thought about it for a while and then tears started running down her cheeks. She said she had just started driving this route and did not know the station well and was scared to get in trouble. I told her I understood. Then she opened the door and apologised to the boy and at last we all could board.

Two hours later, as I was returning to Laguna, there was another bus driver. I sat down when I suddenly heard a voice saying "Hi!" from the opposite side of the isle. It was the boy from the bus station in Laguna. I was happy to see him and asked how he was doing. He told me he was okay but still a bit shaken. He had contacted the head office. I understood it was important to him to have done so. Then he said, "I reacted the way my mother always reacts. I have to change that!" I realised he probably has had to listen to many bitter memories and hurtful experiences from his Afro-American mother. This had become part of him and was triggered in such situations. I smiled and nodded that I understood. He had learned something and got the point, and I was happy. Later that evening I remembered the pigeons that had prepared my subconscious for this happening. Mother Nature had prepared me by giving me help and guidance! What we expect is based on what we have experienced. Our feelings are magnetic. If we choose peace, it also means that we must let go of the old pain story.

We do not see things as they are, we see them as we are.

– Anais Nin

I thought I had truly taken a long time to work on my process of healing. Time is also an illusion, so let us say that I had simply been going through the process. I really had all eternity but still no time to lose. One day I jumped on the train to San Diego, about an hour drive from Laguna. There was an alternative exhibition 'Body, Mind & Spirit Expo' that I wanted to visit. As I waited in the hall, I noticed a group of women standing close by. It seemed we were all waiting for the same lecture that was soon to start. I smiled at them, as that comes easy to me and thankfully here in the States it is not considered something strange or untimely. I simply smile because I am happy. Suddenly a beautiful, tiny, silver haired old lady walked up to me. She had been standing with the group, but now she was beside me for no obvious reason. She didn't greet me, but just smiled and hold my arm as she rested her head on my upper arm. We simply stood there for a while, smiling at each other and it did not seem strange at all. I just allowed it to happen. Then she suddenly with gentle authority said, "You have to let go – now!" That was all she said. I nodded and agreed. And that was it.

I do not think anything happens by coincidence, and that also goes for this free and unconditional 'channelling'. She was right. The universe does not want me to forget this and was giving me a gentle reminder – once again.

Back in Laguna, I am enjoying the beautiful sunshine and everything crossing my path, but suddenly I feel unsettled. Do I really deserve all this? I sat down in a café that I visit frequently and felt great tiredness wash over me. Surprised that I experienced this old feeling again and I was quite sure it had nothing to do with physical exhaustion or unhappiness. All was well on all levels, I thought. But something inside wanted to teach me something more!

I can easily close out the world whenever and wherever I am, so I closed my eyes, settled down and prayed for an answer. I went into my stillness and suddenly I felt the floor becoming a seething whirl pulling me downward. I allowed myself to be led at a neck breaking speed. The bottom of the swirl was of black and brownish dirt. Suddenly it became alive and whispered one simple sentence: 'You have carried too much responsibility!' That was it!

I took a deep breath and was back in the café with my cup of coffee that was still warm. I realised the little grey-haired lady in San Diego was right. I knew mentally I had mostly let go of responsibility for everything that was not mine, but this was at a deeper level. The tiredness was from deep within my cell-memories. It seemed it was rooted in generations before me, or from past incarnations. The cells had not yet let go of these memories. It was an illusion that had gotten stuck. I knew I was not responsible for the choices and pain of others, but my body had not yet been convinced. It still holds on to remembrance.

Arriving home this evening, I settled into a long and deep meditation. I allowed my cells to empty themselves of all thoughts of responsibility for things that really have nothing to do with me. I made it visual as possible as that helps my brain to believe the changes. It passes on the new signals to the cells that create new pathways. I felt better.

The following night I dreamt (Chapter 21: Dream nr 41: Flying on a broom) I was standing outside the house with a group of people. We stood in a line waiting for something. It was a dark night, and we were standing by a lamppost, when one person in the line started to talk with another about me. The comments were negative, and I felt I would at once not take this any longer. Now, I wanted to show them something they really could talk about! I picked up a broom leaning up against the lamppost, mounted it and flew off into the distance, free and laughing!

I woke up laughing out loud. I realised I just had to not care anymore about these tormentors inside and let go of all thoughts about what others believed about me. I had to stop taking everything so personally and seriously. I was reminded Peter Pan only could fly when he had happy thoughts! I had to let go of old beliefs to be 'light enough' to fly away.

When I went to school, they asked me what I wanted to be when I grew up. I wrote down 'happy'. They told me I did not understand the assignment and I told them they did not understand life.

— John Lennon

I will let go of everything and simply breathe in life. Simplicity is the end goal of art. Simplicity is the solution of the genius. But this simplicity is the most difficult for me. I believe to trust is to join this pulse, and rest in the caring togetherness of the great Universe. To just let go and breathe in life. I was told scientists have discovered that human heartbeats naturally synchronize with the pulse of electromagnetic energy the universe emits. I believe to trust is to join this pulse and register the caring togetherness with the great universe – like a baby in mother's womb. Just the thought makes my heartbeat steadier and my breathing calmer.

The next step was not to have any opinion about anything or anybody. I was being told all was as it should be. But I could not rest in this. I needed some control at least over what seemed right and wrong. I feared anarchy. What could I hold on to if no thoughts were right or wrong?

My only option was to get centred, have faith in the Now. My inner guidance and the Source. I could not see other possibilities. I had tried everything else and it did not work.

Think from the end and stay with the source.

– Wayne Dyer

My inner true North Star had led me to sunny Laguna. The collective energy here takes wealth and riches as a given. I understood why I had chosen this place. I was to embrace abundance. I could feel my normally critical attitude slowly melting away. My dreams were calmer, more colorful and stronger.

A good friend of mine in Norway received an enthusiastic email where I described some of the things that were happening. He replied smiling that I had been born with a golden spoon in my mouth. People who know my story know that this is not true. Still, I understood what he meant. I realised this was the energy that I was communicating now. This was not typical of me, but I had dreamed it into existence. Short while back, I would not have been able to do it. I would not have believed I was deserving of any of it. The universe had to work hard to convince me because there had been so much resistance in me.

My mind wants to interpret
All my dreams.
My heart wants to love
All my dreams.
My soul wants to fulfil
All my dreams.

– Sri Chinmoy

The sun was shining and while on my way to the beach I passed a hedge with beautiful red flowers. I felt strong urge to touch them. So, I stopped and held them gently. I could feel the beat of life in them! I sensed my gentle and loving touch was returned by the flowers. Surprised, I a realized a new door had opened for me. We truly are one with all creation. I felt its heartbeat. Nature reveals to us what we need to understand about ourselves.

One day I rented a movie and was sitting on the carpet in my cosy apartment in Laguna Beach watching it when I heard a deep rumble. It was as if a large truck was passing by the house. I thought it strange as no large truck could pass on the small road outside. The rumbling escalated and suddenly the house was lifting as if having been caught by a wave. It was swaying back and forth and up and down before it settled back down again. Yes, I got to experience a California earthquake. It was a big quake. Although it went deep, it only caused ripples on the surface. No damage was done to the house and nothing broke. I was shaken but did not really feel any fear. As soon as I understood what was happening, I attached myself to "a column of light" stretching from the sky through me, down through the centre of the earth, as I prayed to be protected. It was a strange but powerful experience. I was alone but felt completely protected and I had no fear. It was as if the Universe wanted to show me how protected and how truly safe, I really was! As I went to sleep that night, the event was forgotten, and I slept like a baby.

Earthquakes symbolise big and deep changes in life. I imagined seeing pieces of a puzzle shaking around and then falling into place beneath me, as if making sure everything was in the right place for the changes within.

I now felt filled to overflowing with this loving energy and my body was finally starting to heal. The depression I had struggled with before I set out on this journey had vaporised like morning dew in the sun. I felt free and light-hearted as I walked along in the sunshine by the oceanside. Suddenly a tiny bird whizzed overhead. It was so close I could feel the wings against my hair. As I turned around to see what kind of bird it was, I joyfully discovered a hummingbird. It was heading for a green plant on the wall with beautiful flowers. I had never seen a live hummingbird before and now I had even been touched by one!

The hummingbird symbolises great healing power, love, beauty and flexibility. It also stands for refined femininity, subtle consciousness and is extremely sensitive. It is said the flowers love the hummingbird and it is nourished by the sweetest nectar. The hummingbird must be free. If caught, it will die. In the shamanistic wheel of life, the hummingbird is the symbol of the North, which is connected to the elements of air and light. It is told hummingbird passes on wisdom and guidance from our ancestors. How fortunate I was! I have been guided and supported all the way and now I was enjoying the dessert – the honey in my life (Chapter 2: Dream nr 2: Meeting with elephants). The hummingbird's touch confirmed the feelings of joy and love I had received.

My friend Gail, at that time the owner of Art Hotel, was turning sixty and I invited her out for dinner at one of the town's better restaurants. We both ordered, and the conversation was lively.

We were laughing at life's strange turns when the waiter arrived with a free indulgence, he wanted to treat us while we were waiting for the main dish. We were enjoying ourselves immensely when the waiter came back again, this time with a free dessert before our main dish. We giggled happily like two teenagers. As we finished our stay, and I was getting ready to pay, the waiter came to us and said we would get additional 50% discount on the bill. He explained they had so enjoyed having us there.

I was reminded 'when we give, we get in return'. Thankfulness and joy create more of itself. All confirmations and all pleasant experiences are signs from the Universe we are at the right place at the right time. All was well. My sun was shining brightly within me, and my inner gorilla was growing stronger and happier.

The Laws of the Universe work in all areas of our lives and not just on the spiritual plain. It affects all levels. My last project while here in Laguna was to lose weight. I started a strict training program and was training five or six times a week. I was in despair when after three weeks I discovered I had not lost single pound. I complained to my trainer, a beautiful soul. "Do you really believe it will work?" she asked and looked at me with her big, clear eyes. I burst out laughing. Everything suddenly seemed so comical. She was right! I had started the battle against the pounds without really believing I would make it. I had forgotten the body wants cooperation. It is not separated. I should not be fighting against it, but instead should be creating a joyful, working relationships with it.

I had an unconscious expectation this project would not be fun or easy and that's what happened! I thought I had to fight against my extra pounds rather than work with them. My intention concerning my wish to lose some pounds had been blocked as it had not been supported by my emotions. It is comical when we try to do something without believing in it. Without faith, no miracle! Once again, I was reminded that my driving force must be joy and trust. Laughter strengthens the immune system I read somewhere. Humour is conditional to culture, but laughter is universal. It releases, unites and heals.

Chapter 22
The Dream Is Landing

Learn what the magician knows, and it is not magic anymore.

– Richard Bach

I was back at the shaman school, 'The Four Winds', in the desert of California, to join the second part of the training. During one of the breaks I went for a walk in the desert surrounding the site. I liked the solitude there and selected a small height that I wanted to get up on. I wanted to chant on the top of it – if I dared. Looking around I discovered I was alone, so I closed my eyes and turned my face towards the sky. I allowed my voice to flow, strong and free and sensed it carry through all levels and all times – to my ancestors. I have a strong voice and held nothing back. I felt a cleansing power flowing through me, bringing great healing to my heart.

As I stopped and opened my eyes, I discovered two large eagles circling high up – right above me. I greeted them reverently, deeply moved. The eagle is the symbol for 'The Great Spirit' to the Native Americans. I climbed down the hill thankful and overwhelmed to have been honoured by the visit of these two beautiful spirits. I was lost in thought when suddenly my shaman teacher appeared in front of me on the trail. He reached out his arms as if saying 'welcome home' and I accepted the invitation and allowed myself to receive a hug from a warm and strong shaman. The tears were flowing. It was unavoidable. My teacher appeared from nowhere. I was embraced by the power of Mother Earth and the Spirit. How blessed I was.

The more in harmony with yourself you are, the more joyful you are and the more faithful you are. Faith is not to disconnect you from reality – it connects you to reality.

– Paulo Coelho

I was safe and had settled in my own being, accepted myself, my African Sun and my powerful Gorilla who lives in integrity and true power. I was happy and I always laugh much and loudly when I am happy. The sun shines freely and strongly inside of me. *I will not allow for anything to smother it anymore,* I told myself.

I had this dream (Chapter 22: Dream nr 42: Looking into Heaven) the last week at 'The Four Winds'. I dreamt I was lifted high up out in the universe and was able to see into the heavens above me where it was stunningly bright and beautiful and so wonderfully peaceful. Nature was vibrating in colored light, and I heard ethereal music emanating from nature itself. I was filled with intense joy and feeling of freedom. I was hovering somewhere between heaven and earth when I saw down to the earth and realised it also showed up to be a paradise! It was just as lovely and surrounded with the same vibrating colours, joy and beauty as above. And I was part of both worlds!

When I woke, I understood paradise was already on earth! We just do not see it. Our heart is the gate between these two worlds. I awoke with a sparkling joyful and loud laughter. My heart was about to burst from joy. I cannot remember having this feeling before! I could not stop laughing for the rest of the day.

I continually remind myself I still carry with me the "reality" I experienced in this dream. Our hearts are the true portals to this new paradise. We become roadblocks to our own dreams if we do not open our hearts. Everything meets in the heart and all contrast is balanced in the heart. I just had to let it all flow.

There is no way to happiness. Happiness is the way.

– Wayne Dyer

One of the last days at the shaman school, I was on the dusty road between the dormitory and the school building. Kevin, a fellow shaman from Australia, was walking there too. We said a friendly 'hi' as we passed each other on the track. Then I hear him stop. I turn around as he puts down his pack and walks back towards me. He puts his arms around me and holds me close for a long time. I smile and laugh a little embarrassed, and say "Thanks", but he did not let go. We just stood there for a long time. Finally, something loosens up inside of me. I breathe deeply and relax. "That's it." He says with a serious smile he lets go and returns to his backpack. What Kevin did not know was this: I did not really trust men yet. He healed my heart. He certainly is a big shaman with an even bigger heart. I had not been conscious of the fact that I kept my heart closed to men. Kevin showed me what I needed to see. Nothing can be manifested without an open heart. I received and was received.

Happiness and joy result from total acceptance of living in the moment.
— Deepak Chopra

A few days I was scheduled to return to Norway. I took a trip to Santa Monica, on the westside of Los Angeles. I was on my way to a lecture held by Wayne Dyer.

Dr Dyer talked for three hours about living in the moment and living 'without excuses'. He held the lecture without a script because he just wanted to give what he was given there and then. That is how I want to live – without a script!

Afterwards I went out for a bite to eat. It was evening, and the sky was covered with stars, the air was balmy, and the atmosphere was light and happy. It was as if California was showing off by giving me a last wonderful experience before I left for Norway. I found a small, cosy restaurant and sat down to order some food.

While waiting for my dinner, at a small cosy restaurant, I noticed an African woman sitting alone by a table near the window. A stunningly beautiful sight with her hair piled up on top of her head, gracefully holding a glass of wine in her hand. In her African dress, she was like a queen. I was fascinated by this woman with her beautiful posture, head held high, gazing straight ahead of her as if to tell the world she belonged there. I was very moved and would have loved to paint her.

This beautiful and proud African woman and I were both out travelling the world. Our lives were blooming because of the freedom in our hearts.

ဂ ဂ ဂ ဂ ဂ

"What now?" They asked me when I returned to Norway. Yes, what now? I asked myself and knew the answer did not really matter.

It was autumn in Norway, and I was sitting with a group of friends when a young man who I did not really know, addressed me and asked what I had been doing that summer. Before I was even able to reply he said wryly, "Don't say that you have been lying in the meadow with a good book and listened to the grass growing." I burst out laughing because that was exactly what I had been doing! I laughed so hard tears rolled down my cheeks. Of course I spotted the sarcasm. It reminded me I was in Norway now. I could not stop laughing. They did not understand my choices had been made from love of myself. I had peace in my heart and the freedom to dream a new life into being.

I sold my home to set out travelling, to discover who I truly am. This does not mean everyone must do the same. It simply means we choose what gives us joy. Maybe that is what we most fear: to let go, take a chance and allow ourselves to be guided.

My dreams revealed what I needed to see and helped me to confront and release the pain story from my past.

I give thanks to my dreams.

We all make our choices based either on fear or love. I look at how I have been supported and guided through all my journey and how I have received a rainbow of gifts and experiences by choosing love over fear.

I believe I am ready to fly now. I am grounded in my heart and Mother Earth. The universe is on my side. How can I fail? I am no longer scared of the waves it might cause, nor am I afraid of the light within. I have experienced the truth of the saying, It's better to light a candle than to curse the darkness. With childlike faith I look up at the stars and ask for guidance and support. I have regained my trust in this earthly life.

I know I must step carefully and respect everyone's journey. And also I must love and respect my own path of life. My inner work is as important as my outer work. The conflict between outside pressure to succeed and the inner desire for peace, harmony and beauty had once left me ill. My desert-walks and the time spent in quiet, and growth woke me up and healed me. I am guided and supported to live this new awareness – with integrity and joy.

Now I have unwrapped my inner Sun and greet it every morning as I welcome the day. I anchor my awareness to this quiet, warm and strong source within my Self. With this safe connection and support, I freely fly.

Sources of Inspirations

I have been helped and nourished by the work of many wise healers, authors and guides.

They all supported me in awakening my own slumbering wisdom.

A small book, *The Warrior of the Light,* by Paulo Coelho, has accompanied me on the journey and supplied me with daily, small, nourishing mouthfuls.

Wayne Dyer's books also inspired me and gave a practical humane view of life's small and large challenges.

Neal Donald Walsch is one of the great spiritual authors of our time. His story and work has inspired and awakened me.

Alberto Villoldo is an anthroposophist, professor, shaman, author and the founder of the shaman school, *The Four Winds*. I was lucky to be a student of this healing energy teaching and the teachings the oneness that we are all part of.

Sandra Ingerman, author and shaman gave me a unique approach to the great mystic within through her book, *Soul Retrieval.*

Robert Moss, the author of *Active Dreaming*, is a conveyer of modern shamanism and dream work, and I have learned a lot from his books.

Deepak Chopra's books have also been a great inspiration in my awakening. I realised no one must give up their faith, in accepting and loving each other across culture and religion.

Jerry and Esther Hicks books have opened the universe to me. They contain an amazing amount of information and guidance regarding the laws of the universe, channelled from the soul group called Abraham.

Marianne Williamson, author, healer and lecturer, was one of the first people who woke me up to the importance of self-development and awareness. Her book 'Return to Love', among others, has had great influence on me.

Author and shaman, Serge K. King, researched the different shamanistic cultures of the world and describes the Hawaiian shaman tradition as the most unconditional, loving and peaceful of them all.

Benedicte Thiis and her illustrated book, *Regnbuetreet* (The Rainbow tree) gave me a foundation in interpreting symbols.

Author and shaman Don Miguel Ruiz and his easily presented little books have taught me a lot.

The medium and author James Van Praagh has also made an impression in my life with his wise and caring disseminations.

Echart Tolle gave the world *The Power of Now,* that really opened my awareness. His teaching gave me deeper insight in my heart.

Barbel Mohr, the author of the book, *Cosmic Ordering*, gives strong and clear guidance regarding our road onward.

Gary R. Renard taught me about the power and mystery of forgiveness in his book *Love Has Forgotten No One: The Answer to Life.*

Gill Edwards works became especially important to me in understanding and working with diseases.

Lastly, I want to thank Ailo Gaup, who recently left this earth. He was a Norwegian shaman and the author of *Sjamansonen* (Shaman Zone). His early encouragement and interest in this book made me feel acknowledged and was important to this book becoming the reality in your hand.

There are so many books I could recommend but I must limit it and simply give a great thanks to the universe for leading me to these wise teachers.

Index of the Dreams

All dreams need to be interpreted in relation to the situation and the emotional state of the dreamer. The dream is often a comment or some advice to your current situation in your life. That is why my story needs to be told for my dreams to be relevant. That is how it works for you too. My own interpretations are also based on my experiences and feelings toward the symbols occurring in my dreams. Many symbols are archetypal and universal and that need to be incorporated in our interpretations. Maybe that will inspire you to study more of this old knowledge.

If the dream is about something scary, its purpose is not to scare but to remind you of your own fear. For example, the snake is not appearing in your dream to scare you, but to remind you of the medicine this symbol stands for; That is about transformation and shedding you skin, your old story that you identify with, and that you no longer have any use for. It can feel scary to let go.

Our dreams are our inner knowledge trying to guide us.

Index